'A good basic textbook for both students and those with many years of experience. It is readable, easy to understand, and contains a number of practical teaching examples. If I was starting out in the caring profession I would buy this book.'

Barbara Coleman, BA. MA. MTh. M.Phil. SRN, SCM, HV Cert. HV Tutor Cert.
Cert. Ed. Cert. of Christian Studies. Cert. of Higher Education in Theology.
Cert. of Christian Counselling. Staff Tutor in Theology, Chester
University for Ordinands and Reader training

'As a nurse with 25 years of experience, and as a student of counselling, I found the book extremely useful for expanding my knowledge on this vast subject. The examples offered throughout the text make the reading easy and very enjoyable. I recommend this volume to students and professionals, as I am sure all readers will be able to apply some of the acquired knowledge into their professional practice, as well as into their personal life.'

Daniela Cismasu, LLB, Dip. Nursing, Dip Hypnotherapy

'I really enjoyed the book and learnt about some interesting aspects of practice. The book discusses intersectionality, and this is so important. Intersectionality should be covered on training for all the professions. I also liked the balance between academic theories, questions for reflection and practical advice. I would have loved this book to be in my college library when I was training. It's useful to think about the distinctions and overlaps between the helping professions, and how we can communicate more clearly.'

Elizabeth Cartwright, BA (Hons) French and Latin, PGCE
Primary Education, Professional Diploma in Integrative
Counselling and Psychotherapy

'Communication and interviewing skills are key building blocks to social work, counselling and the helping professions more broadly. This book aims to deal with these important issues for practice and does so in an accessible way.'

Professor Di Bailey Division Leader, Social Work and Health,
Associate Dean for Research, School of Social Sciences,
Nottingham Trent University

'This book could not come at a better time. Professor Higham has drawn on both stalwart and contemporary theories of communication and brought them into excellent utility for practice. This book that leaves no form of communication unturned, is accessible, informative and recommended as a staple for learners but also a reminder for all of us no matter where our starting point.'

Dr. Trish Hafford-Letchfield, Professor of Social Care,
Middlesex University

'This book provides an access route for developing practice, written in language for both the emerging and experienced practitioner. It covers the basic principles and wider spectrum of essential knowledge and awareness of self for communication and interviewing skills. A useful tool for reflection in supervision.'

Communication and Interviewing Skills for Practice in Social Work, Counselling and the Health Professions

This book supports and develops the communication and interviewing skills of professional practitioners and student practitioners in social work, counselling, and the health professions.

Combining work on personal and social constructs, the search for meaning, and ecological theory, this book both provides an integrated discussion of practice and presents a balanced approach when discussing psychological, biological, and social influences on individual well-being. Furthermore, it emphasises the influence of social contexts on behaviour and well-being, as well as valuing and encouraging the application of practitioners' prior experience and learning (APEL) to new knowledge and understanding. Containing a range of practice examples to stimulate learning, this book promotes a collaboration between the professions, and welcomes the contributions of people who use services, patients, and clients.

Communication and Interviewing Skills for Practice in Social Work, Counselling and the Health Professions will be of interest to all undergraduate and postgraduate social work students, as well as new and experienced professional health care practitioners.

Patricia Higham is a registered social worker and counsellor, and served as a non-executive director and lay member of NHS organisations in Nottinghamshire. She completed a BA degree at Wellesley College in Massachusetts, a postgraduate social work qualification at the University of Sheffield, a PhD at Cranfield University, and a part-time counselling qualification over a three-year period. She is Professor of Social Work (Emeritus) at Nottingham Trent University. She worked part-time for the Quality Assurance Agency, Skills for Care, DeMontfort University, and for the Health and Care Professions Council. Her experience includes statutory social work in Sheffield, Milton Keynes, Northamptonshire, and mental health outreach in a rural area of Pennsylvania, USA. She is a life member of the British Association of Social Workers and a member of the National Association of Social Workers, USA. She is a member of the British Association of Counselling and Psychotherapy. She volunteers as a counsellor two days a week for charities that support women who experience domestic violence.

Student Social Work

This exciting new textbook series is ideal for all students studying to be qualified social workers, whether at undergraduate or masters level. Covering key elements of the social work curriculum, the books are accessible, interactive and thought-provoking.

New titles

Social Work and Social Policy, 2nd ed.
An Introduction
Jonathan Dickens

Mental Health Social Work in Context 2nd ed.
Nick Gould

Social Work in a Changing Scotland
Edited by Viviene E. Cree and Mark Smith

Social Theory for Social Work
Ideas and Applications
Christopher Thorpe

Human Growth and Development
An Introduction for Social Workers 2nd Edition
John Sudbery and Andrew Whittaker

Counselling Skills for Social Workers
Hilda Loughran

Social Work and Integrated Care
Robin Miller

Communication and Interviewing Skills for Practice in Social Work, Counselling and the Health Professions
Patricia Higham

https://www.routledge.com/Student-Social-Work/book-series/SSW

Communication and Interviewing Skills for Practice in Social Work, Counselling and the Health Professions

Patricia Higham

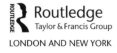
Routledge
Taylor & Francis Group

LONDON AND NEW YORK

First published 2020
by Routledge
2 Park Square, Milton Park, Abingdon, Oxon OX14 4RN

and by Routledge
52 Vanderbilt Avenue, New York, NY 10017

Routledge is an imprint of the Taylor & Francis Group, an informa business

British Library Cataloguing in Publication Data
A catalogue record for this book is available from the British Library

Library of Congress Cataloging-in-Publication Data
A catalog record has been requested for this book

ISBN: 978-1-138-34293-4 (hbk)
ISBN: 978-1-138-34294-1 (pbk)
ISBN: 978-0-429-43949-0 (ebk)

Typeset in Bembo
by Taylor & Francis Books

This book is dedicated to the Rev. Canon Jack Higham (1933–2018) for his support and encouragement.

Contents

Illustrations

Figures

Tables

Acknowledgements

Whilst writing this book, I have welcomed and benefited from the comments, suggestions, and support of professional practitioners, users of services, colleagues, and friends; and I have welcomed the warm support of my sons, Hugh Higham and Tim Higham.

Chapter 1

Introducing Communication and Interviewing Skills

Introduction

Communication and Interviewing Skills for Practice in Social Work, Counselling and the Health Professions is written for professional practitioners and students to help them develop their professional awareness, essential practice skills, and strengthen their knowledge, understanding and expertise for using communication and interviewing skills in their practice. A confident grasp of flexible communication and interviewing skills is fundamental to good practice. Without appropriate communication, practitioners in a range of professions will not be able to develop effective relationships with colleagues and with the people they are trying to help – clients, people who use services and patients – and without effective relationships, they will be unable to select, combine, and use communication theories appropriately. Whilst it is helpful to be familiar with a range of theories, current research, legislation and policies, these kinds of knowledge are not sufficient on their own to ensure good practice. Communication and interviewing skills are 'bread and butter' tools that guide and sustain practice. Communication and interviewing skills are not meant to be fixed entities; they have to adapt to contemporary contexts that present new dilemmas and they have to support new intervention strategies. Being open to new techniques will enable practitioners to continue effective practice. Practitioners who wish to keep their skills up-to-date will select new technological communication tools, as well as using tried and tested communication strategies. Those who pride themselves on being up-to-date practitioners will engage with new dilemmas and use new techniques in a spirit of enquiry, without pre-judging people or situations. Confident use of communication and interviewing skills will ease the path towards mastery of new practice strategies.

Whilst writing this book, I considered my current and previous experience and drew on my practice knowledge of social work and counselling, my knowledge of the health professions, the contributions of professional colleagues, and the voices of persons who receive professional services. I reflected on my experience of university teaching, management, and quality assurance, my learning and experience as a counsellor, my volunteer experience as a board member and chair of different charities; my experiences of participatory research; and my personal, professional, and organisational relationships. These experiences provided the grounding for my practice, but as well as looking back and reflecting on my previous experiences, I also try to remain open to learning new strategies that might help to resolve contemporary dilemmas. This book has been written in that spirit of looking back, reviewing previous knowledge and understanding, but being open to new kinds of issues. Readers will make best use of the book by reflecting on what they have learned previously, and identifying knowledge and skills they want to acquire for their future practice.

Drawing on literature and research

The book draws on relevant literature and research, and adopts a historical approach that features classic writers who have shaped professional practice, as well as recent authors' research and reflections. Readers will recognise some texts which influenced generations of practitioners, but the classic texts are not presented as the 'last word' of a particular concept or theory. Instead, these texts can offer a helpful starting point for the reader to recognise classic theories of practice that made a difference, and the ways newer perceptions and issues continue to modify the classic theories. The classic texts provide building blocks for new ideas, and sometimes prompt a powerful reaction – a turn of ideas towards different practice directions. When I mention a classic text, I expect readers to value the historic relevance of ideas that have influenced professional practice, and to explore how these ideas have changed over the years. These classic ideas will be considered within the context of contemporary social policy and events that exert powerful influences on our lives. Sometimes a classic idea for practice is reiterated and expressed somewhat differently by a contemporary writer. For example, Rowan (2016) stresses the importance of 'listening with the fourth ear' – building on Reik's concept of 'listening with the third ear' (1983) – and explaining that the practitioner must take note of an individual's social contexts and find out about the environmental issues that the individual experienced in the past and experiences in the present day. Although different theoretical concepts are presented initially in a linear fashion – one at a time – as the book progresses, an astute reader will experience growing awareness of the links between the separate concepts.

Integrating knowledge and skills in practice

The skilled practitioner not only looks back but considers new theories and strategies for practice, and asks the question 'how do I put it all together – integrate the different theories and techniques?' It is my belief that practitioners need to learn how to integrate different kinds of knowledge and skills within their practice. As discussed previously, they first learn how to do this by becoming familiar with particular skills and particular kinds of knowledge in a linear, separate process. For example, they may read a book that promotes the person-centred approach to communication (Rogers, 1961) and then read other publications that promote a behavioural approach to communication (Beck, 2011; Ellis, 2008), and then a third publication that advocates a psychodynamic approach (Freud, 1986). They may take short courses to learn new techniques and approaches to communication and interviewing.

How can a professional practitioner choose which approach or approaches to adopt? Sometimes they are attracted to a particular approach and they may then decide to adopt that approach – they may subsequently declare 'I am a person-centred' practitioner or 'psychodynamic' or 'cognitive-behavioural'. But practice itself is not always so neat and tidy. Quite often, a practitioner may recognise that it is not appropriate to use just one approach – one size does not fit all! The practitioner may find that tools for practice –

theory and methods – must be selected, modified, and combined in a very individual way to communicate with a specific individual. Confident use of communication skills will provide you with appropriate strategies for putting your chosen theories and methods into practice.

The book will explore the dilemmas of choosing a particular approach for a particular person who seeks help for a particular issue, and will argue that a practitioner's choices require not only deepening theoretical knowledge, but also acquiring *practice wisdom* and learning how to exercise *professional judgement.*

Practice wisdom and professional judgement

Both of these concepts – *practice wisdom* and *professional judgement* – rely on the acquisition and exercise of intuitive knowledge that a practitioner instinctively uses to underpin their practice decisions. *Practice wisdom* is an internal reservoir of knowledge, accrued through a discerning selection of theory and methods, further study, practice experience, reflection and supervision. These processes help a practitioner build the mental agility for effective practice. *Professional judgement* is the practitioner's inner mental process for making practice decisions that impact people's lives. Acquiring professional wisdom and exercising professional judgement are concepts that are closely related to each other.

As a practitioner acquires practice experience, learns to reflect critically on their practice, undertakes regular continuing professional development, and brings issues and questions to professional supervision, they will begin to use their accumulated experience with increasing confidence. The ways that individual practitioners make their professional judgements and develop practice wisdom are strongly influenced by professional codes of ethics (particularly when a particular professional decision might, for example, result in removing a child from their parents or in compulsorily admitting an individual to hospital for mental health treatment). The practitioner exercises professional wisdom and professional judgement not only when making life-changing recommendations and exercising statutory power, but also when maintaining professional relationships on a day-to-day basis.

The importance of personal and social contexts

Personal and professional experience shape a practitioner's choice of theories and methods. My professional and personal background has influenced my belief in the value of personal and social contexts. To give an example of the importance of personal and social contexts, consider how a psychologist, after examining a patient, may categorise a patient with a diagnosis of OCD (obsessive-compulsive disorder). Whilst accepting that this diagnosis is valid, I should want to look further (but sensitively) at how an individual has lived their life in the past and lives in the present day, and explore how their personal and social contexts contribute to their present awareness of their situation. I would bear in mind that getting to know an individual is a gradual process that is sustained by efforts to build a warm, trusting relationship. I would try, in a non-intrusive way, to discover whether the person can recall their childhood, what kind of memories they carry forward into their adult lives, how they remember their school days – either with recollections of their friends, or with memories of being bullied by others. Do they remember experiences of poverty, abuse, deprivation, and/or separation from parents? Do they continue to experience poverty and abuse in the present day? Were they in the care of a local authority as a child? What kinds of jobs did/do they do? Were they ever homeless? What are their underlying beliefs and values about themselves and others? I argue that it is important to learn about an individual's personal and social contexts – the events in their lives that shape who they are – before making a professional judgement.

Constructing and reconstructing meaning

Communicating with people means that you must listen carefully to what they say and encourage them to share their personal stories or narratives, at the same time informing them of the ethical boundaries of confidentiality. As you listen, you will become aware that individuals construct and reconstruct their memories of events and the meanings of their relationships and experiences (Kelly, 1955; Neimeyer, 2009; 2001). This is not being dishonest; it is a search for meaning, trying to make sense of what has happened (Frankl, 2011, 1969). A professional practitioner will value the importance of constructing and reconstructing meaning, and will learn to use their communication skills to increase understanding and build trust to encourage individuals to share their stories.

The voices of Experts by Experience

Most importantly, in this book I have tried to listen to the voices of persons and practitioners. One of the most powerful movements that brought change to the caring professions over the last thirty years is the rise of 'Experts by Experience' – the clients, patients, and users of services. Over the years, the voices of 'Experts by Experience' have grown stronger and more numerous, so that their voices now exert an influence on how services are planned, delivered, and experienced. Professional practitioners now recognise (or should recognise) that good practice depends on listening to the experiences of service users/patients/clients and their carers. Their feedback on their experiences – both good and bad – of how the 'caring services' respond to their needs is an essential building block of good practice.

Objectives

The book's objectives are to enable:

- social work, counselling and health professions students to develop their communication and interviewing skills
- experienced social workers, counsellors, and health practitioners to integrate communication and interviewing skills within their professional practice

Both practitioners and students will learn to

- listen to the voices of 'Experts by Experience' and their carers
- use personal and social contexts to enhance their professional judgement
- value the importance of constructing and reconstructing meaning
- develop practice wisdom relevant to their profession
- apply communication and interviewing skills within multi-professional contexts

Who this book is for

The content is relevant to two audiences: qualifying students in social work, counselling, and the health professions, and experienced practitioners of those professions. These two audiences will use the book in different ways. This book will support your practice, whether you read it as a beginning practitioner or as an experienced practitioner.

- If you are a student on a qualifying professional course, you will learn to adopt a systematic approach to learning with a clear understanding of links between theory and practice – a 'how to' approach. You will study the book's contents to take essential beginning steps towards acquiring professional expertise.
- If you are an experienced practitioner, you will want to review and reconsider your reasons for selecting and combining different practice approaches. You will draw on the book's contents to enhance your ability to adapt and integrate aspects of effective communication and interviewing within your practice.
- This book will help you, whether you are a beginning or an experienced practitioner, to learn, review, and develop your own individual distinctive approach.

Looking beyond professional boundaries

The book explores the commonalities and differences of how communication and interviewing skills are used within a number of professions. These skills are not practised exclusively or 'owned' by any one of the professions. Each profession has its own distinctive role and purpose, and uses its communication and interviewing skills within practice situations and outcomes that differ from those of other professions. Taking these differences into account, the book offers practice examples from a range of professional and occupational settings. Although the book's focus is on social work, counselling and the health professions, the audience of readers can extend to staff in other helping environments, for example, housing associations, children's centres, and educational and community organisations.

Key themes

Key themes provide a conceptual basis for understanding communication and interviewing in particular practice situations. These include how:

- practitioners can integrate their practice skills

  A complex mix of social, psychological, and contextual influences on behaviour and well-being provides a framework for practising communication and interviewing skills. The framework integrates separate components of *the person who uses services + the practitioner + the particular issue + ethical considerations + context + methods and approaches*. These components are present within every unique professional situation that involves communication and interviewing skills.

- practitioners communicate within multi-*professional contexts*

Professional practitioners who practise in multi-professional teams learn to liaise with each other across professional boundaries. In multi-professional practice, different professions use communication and interviewing skills both jointly and separately. The book will attempt to build a shared understanding of how practitioners can communicate across their professional boundaries and build practice that is inter-professional.

- *information-giving* is essential to professional communication

Practitioners need to provide clear accurate verbal and written information in their communication with colleagues, other professional practitioners, and most of all, with people who are at the receiving end of communication and interviewing processes.

- *social and personal contexts* and the *search for meaning* influence communication

A contemporary theoretical basis for practising interviewing and communication skills recognises the importance of personal and social construct theories (Kelly, 1955; Neimeyer, 2009, 2001), Frankl's search for meaning (2014, 2011, 1969), and Bronfenbrenner's ecological theory (1979) as key concepts.

- *patient/service user/client groups* modify the use of professional power in communication

Each profession is now expected to take note of the views and feedback of persons who use services. Their participation modifies the dominance of professional power.

- *situations of loss* and *crisis* raise important communication issues for practitioners

Loss is a familiar concept with a broad application. Feelings of loss and crisis arise when someone dies, when a treasured object goes missing, or when illness impairs health and well-being, to give some examples. Practitioners should recognise and respond appropriately to these feelings and attempt to learn a range of theoretical interpretations of loss and mourning.

- practitioners' *prior learning and experience,* and *continuing professional development* deepen their awareness and skills.

Practitioners are encouraged to apply their relevant learning and experience to new knowledge and understanding. Communication and interviewing are life skills, developed from childhood onwards, not introduced for the first time when learning how to be a professional practitioner. Prior achievements and experiences impact on how new learning is received and used. New learning from experience and from continuing professional development activities expands understanding and confidence.

The book aims to increase practitioners' commitment to continuing professional development and sustaining excellent practice. Ongoing professional development is not optional, but is necessary for ensuring that practice is up-to-date. Professional practitioners continue to learn through reflecting on experience, thinking about their practice, peer discussion, reading, and professional supervision, as well as through formal learning. Continuing professional development helps to build practice wisdom and develop advanced skills in communicating and interviewing.

How the book is organised

The nineteen chapters discuss selected theoretical and methodological approaches and provide practice examples of how to combine different approaches within particular situations with particular individuals. Successive chapters introduce and reiterate key themes.

- This first chapter (Chapter 1) introduces the book's objectives, key themes and organisational structure, and establishes that the book is intended for professional practitioners and students of social work, counselling and the health professions.
- Chapter 2 focuses on *persons who receive services*. Each profession uses different terminology to describe a person who is at the receiving end of a professional communication (who may be called a 'client', 'patient', 'service user' or other designation). *Please note that these designations are used inter-changeably throughout the book.* Chapter 2 considers the contributions of service users who are *Experts by Experience* (Beresford, 2016); the concept of intersectionality (Collins and Bilge, 2016); the first steps towards effective communication; phases of communication; the significance of social contexts, and the importance of shared humanity.
- Chapter 3 discusses professional practitioners and their roles, and how persons who receive services perceive the different helping professions. Service users' social contexts affect their communication with practitioners. Similarities and differences in communication styles are explained, as also how changing service delivery contexts influence communication styles. A *paternalistic model*, a *medical model*, a *social model*, and a *participatory* model pursue different methods of communication. These different models ebb and flow in popularity. Therapeutic relationships, rapport and empathy are important aspects of professional communication; and comprise essential skills for professional communication.
- Chapter 4 discusses a range of communication approaches, advising practitioners to choose approaches that suit the purpose of the communication (either formal and informal) and the person who receives the communication; to select compatible theoretical methods and develop a personal style aligned with the values of their profession and the purposes of their employing organisation; to consider how professional status and power influence communication; and whether persons at the receiving end of a professional communication always understand its intended meaning. Patient/service user/client groups have changed the nature of professional communication, encouraging practitioners to listen to the views of people who use services, and diminishing the impact of professional power on communication and interviewing. The *head/mind/reason* approach to communication is contrasted with the *heart/soul/emotions* approach, which includes the use of *relationships* (Biestek, 1992, 1957), the *use of self* (Dewane, 2006), and the *art of practice* (England, 1986).
- Chapter 5 explores interviewing as a form of communication, conducted with different styles to achieve different purposes; communication skills and processes for conducting an interview, and conversely, skills and processes when the practitioner is

the interviewee; interviewing within the context of professional power structures; and how equal opportunities legislation and the contributions of patient/service user/client/carer groups modify these structures.

- Chapter 6 discusses conceptual themes that provide a basis for communicating and interviewing in particular practice situations. These include how *social and personal contexts* influence communication; listening with the 'fourth ear', how practitioners and clients/service users/carers/patients *search for meaning*; how meaning is *constructed and re-constructed* according to an individual's emotional needs and life events; and how *cognitive approaches* assist with communication.
- Chapter 7 discusses information giving as a means of communication. The practitioner should avoid confusing 'information giving' with 'giving advice'. Information giving has the potential to provide an individual with strategies and sources of help that enable them to tackle their problems themselves. Information-giving promotes choice, rather than being dictatorial and over-authoritarian. For individuals who grew up with authoritarian critical parents, and who experienced authoritarian regimes at school and at work, *information-giving* can build confidence about how to resolve their problems. The growth of supportive group work programmes about assertiveness, domestic violence, and parenting skills helps service users to acquire skills and gain confidence.
- Chapter 8 discusses how ethical concerns shape communication and interviewing skills; how the concerns of people who use services influence communication; *intersectionality* as an ethical concern; how information empowers but may pose ethical risks; how ethical codes change in response to public concerns, and how professional judgement guides decision-making when ethical issues raise major concerns.
- Chapter 9 explores how organisations use communication and interviewing skills in different ways and for different purposes, and discusses communicating effectively across professional boundaries and valuing each profession's contributions. Communicating across the professional boundaries of separate professions is now a necessary skill for multi-professional practice. Perspectives of different professions and different roles can be biased. The chapter questions whether the separate professions value each other's contributions, and whether practice is diminished if they persistently doubt the value of working with other professions.
- Chapter 10 discusses communicating with technology, computers, and artificial intelligence, and how logarithms can both help and hinder good communication. The chapter explores issues of hidden power and control that may unwittingly accompany the spread of artificial intelligence, including how the use of logarithms to predict behaviour may be flawed because prejudicial attitudes (racism, sexism) may be embedded in the researched data used to construct the logarithm.
- Chapter 11 discusses communication in different practice settings, presenting additional theories, methods, and approaches for effective communication and interviewing that depend on good communication skills and multi-professional practice. The chapter discusses practising in crisis situations; and engaging with persons with a mental illness, diabetes, addictions, or obesity.
- Chapter 12 discusses how practitioners can communicate effectively with people who face situations of loss. Classic theories that underpin our understanding of how to deal with the stress of loss are explored and evaluated for their effectiveness in

contemporary communities. The chapter discusses different kinds of loss: loved ones who die or who are no longer living nearby, the loss of relationships, belief, employment, physical capacity, and financial security, and how practitioners can help grieving individuals.

- Chapter 13 discusses how domestic violence affects communication. Identifying domestic violence and authoritarian control as problems within family relationships is relatively recent, and is linked with the rise of the feminist movement. Society is no longer able to turn a blind eye to the physical and mental abuse experienced by individuals who are involved in intimate relationships. The chapter explores how the impact of domestic violence causes the victim of violence to 'freeze', to feel afraid, and to be mistrustful. Communication with a frightened individual is not easy. Trust is hard won. The chapter explores how group communication can help to build confidence and break down barriers, and how individual practitioners must be honest about the extent of their own power and authority over the abused individual.

- Chapter 14 discusses how meaning is constructed by using life stories and biographical approaches as a means of communication. Social workers have used this approach with children in care to prepare the children for adoptive placements, but the book argues that life stories and biographical approaches can be therapeutic practice tools with adults who have experienced turbulent lives. The user of services and the professional practitioner can communicate together in a collaborative way to build the life story, and then write down the story. This method of communication can reveal how individuals develop certain beliefs – 'constructions' about themselves and the events in their lives.

- Chapter 15 discusses communication with older people. Despite Western society's growing awareness that older people are an increasing part of the population, their voices are not heard sufficiently to change society's over-all biased perception of old age as only decrepitude, problems, and neediness. Whilst some older people depend on health and social care services to maintain their well-being, others lead independent lives. Communication with older people, however, is dominated by ageist assumptions. Communication is dominated by questions about health, mobility, medication, loss, etc. The prior assumption is that old age is dreadful and beset with problems. Older people are assumed to be helpless, like children. This chapter explores how communication with older people can avoid stereotypical negative assumptions about old age.

- Chapter 16 explores some of the issues a professional practitioner should consider when communicating with people with a physical impairment, a learning difficulty, or a mental health issue. Some of these conditions are life long and others are acquired later in life through progressive diseases or accidents. The professional practitioner's communication skills must convey acceptance and encouragement, and engage with the individual effectively, recognising that they are Experts by Experience.

- Chapter 17 explores present-day concerns about children and young people, as well as traditional attitudes that denied children legal rights, education and institutionalised them when their parents were unable to care for them. Gradual reform of children's services has led to improvements in authoritarian regimes. Present-day communication with children and young people requires specialist practitioner skills.

Communication helps children and young people, particularly those who are in care, to acquire knowledge of the forgotten events of their lives. It is hoped that a new emphasis on relationship-based practice will lead to a less overtly authoritarian approach to communicating with children and young people.

- Chapter 18 discusses how to take responsibility for your professional development and improve your communication and interviewing skills by reflecting on your prior learning and experience and becoming aware of how these contribute to your current practice; undertaking selected formal professional development activities; personally evaluating your practice experience to identify your strengths and weaknesses; and by remembering the importance of *self-care* to prevent yourself from becoming emotionally and physically over-fatigued. The messages in this chapter are for professional practitioners who define themselves as professionals who are motivated to continually question and improve their practice by adhering to their profession's ethical standards, receiving appropriate professional supervision, and by not being afraid to modify their techniques when asked.
- Chapter 19 summarises the book's content and main themes, and encourages practitioners to continue to develop their communication and interviewing skills. The main points of each chapter are summarised in this final chapter, and the reader is encouraged to embark on a life-long journey of further development of their skills and knowledge.

Some final considerations about the purposes of the book

The book's contents represent my discoveries and reflections so far. I have learned much whilst writing this book, and I shall continue to discover and promote effective communication and interviewing skills. I hope the same will be true for readers of the book. My thanks are offered to the individuals who shared their experiences, listened to my ideas, and helped me to increase my understanding. I welcome readers' feedback and suggestions, so that learning can continue.

References

Beck, Judith S., with Beck, Aaron (2011) *Cognitive Behavioral Therapy, Basics and Beyond*. The Guildford Press: New York.

Beresford, P. (2016) *All Our Welfare: Towards Participatory Social Policy*. Policy Press: London.

Biestek, F. (1992, 1957) *The Casework Relationship*. Routledge: London.

Bronfenbrenner, U. (1979) *The Ecology of Human Developmenti*. Harvard University Press: Cambridge, MA.

Collins, Patricia Hill, and Bilge, Sirma (2016) *Intersectionality*. Polity Press: Cambridge.

Dewane, Claudia J. (2006) 'Use of self: a primer revisited', *Clinical Social Work Journal*, 34(4). Winter, pp. 543–558.

Ellis, Albert, with Abrams, M. and Abrams, L. (2008) *Theories of Personality: Critical Perspectives*. Sage: New York.

England, Hugh (1986) *Social Work As Art: Making Sense for Good Practice*. Allen & Unwin: London.

Frankl, V. (2014) *The Will to Meaning: Foundations and Applications of Logotherapy*. Meridian: London.

Freud, S. (1986 edition) *The Essentials of Psycho-Analysis* (selected by Anna Freud). Penguin: London.

Frankl, V. (2011, 1969) *Man's Search for Ultimate Meaning*. Basic Books: Cambridge, MA.

Kelly, G.A. (1955*) The Psychology of Personal Constructs*. Routledge: New York.

Neimeyer, Robert A. (2001) (ed.) *Meaning Reconstruction and the Experience of Loss*. American Psychological Association: Washington, D. C., pp. 1–9.

Neimeyer, Robert A. (2009) *Constructivist Psychotherapy*. Routledge: London.

Reik, Theodor (1983) *Listening with the Third Ear: The Inner Experience of a Psychoanalyst*. Farrar Strauss and Giroux: New York.

Rogers, C. R. (1961) *On Becoming a Person*. Constable: London.

Rowan, John (2016) *The Reality Game: A Guide to Humanistic Counselling and Psychotherapy*. 3rd Edition. Routledge: Abingdon.

Samson, Patricia L. (2014) 'Practice wisdom: the art and science of social work', *Journal of Social Work Practice*. Volume 29, Issue 2, pp. 119–131. Taylor and Francis: London.

Taylor, B. and Whittaker, A. (2018) 'Professional judgement and decision making in social work', *Journal of Social Work Practice*. Volume 32. pp. 105–109. Taylor and Francis: London.

Chapter 2

The person who receives services

Who is the person? Different professional designations

How do different professions designate the *'person'?* Each profession uses different terminology to describe a person who receives a professional communication. Currently, social workers tend to use 'person who uses services' or 'service user'; counsellors will use 'client'; and health practitioners will use the term 'patient'. Different designations link the person with the service that is being offered. These designations change over time, as services seek to adopt more non-stigmatising language.

The variety of designations across the professions suggests that each profession holds a different perspective of a person. Perhaps the training for a specific profession results in a practitioner perceiving only part of a person, rather than the person as a whole. The entirety of an individual person is complex, puzzling, and difficult to comprehend. Communication that comprehends the whole of a person is more difficult to achieve than professionals may anticipate. Service user and patient groups, sometimes called *Experts by Experience* (Beresford, 2016**)**, who contribute to service planning and evaluation, can help professionals see, hear, and understand the 'whole person' who receives services. Above all, this person is a human being whose designation as *client, person who uses services*, or *patient* should not obscure a practitioner's perception of the person's humanity. Enabling *Experts by Experience* to inform professional practitioners of the economic and social realities that impact on clients' lives is an example of a good partnership that supports more logical decision-making.

Intersectionality

The impact of *intersectionality* – a concept that describes the inter-connections between race, class, disability, gender, disadvantage, and stigma (Collins and Bilge, 2016) – is intended to build mutual understanding and acceptance of a range of stigmatised identities. Intersectionality originated as a feminist concept that portrayed how certain structural and political aspects of personhood can affect the nature of communication. The early days of the feminist movement – 'the first wave' – unwittingly promoted an unacknowledged assumption that all women were apt to experience the same inequalities in their lives. White middle-class women dominated the feminist movement, which was not, at that point, truly representative of women from ethnic minorities, women who were poor, disabled, lesbian, trans-sexual, and who lacked education. 'First wave' feminism initially did not acknowledge these women and give them a voice, or recognise the complexities of their disadvantaged situations.

Once these omissions were fully recognised, the door was opened to developing a much broader understanding of disadvantage – that many disadvantages and inequalities with different characteristics were inter-connected – hence the term intersectionality to describe the inter-relationships. Two black women in the USA began to study the inter-relationship between a having a female identity and being a member of an ethnic minority. Kimberlé Crenshaw (1989) was the first person to write about the connected nature of disadvantage and increase the public's awareness of these inequalities. Patricia Hill Collins (1990) then expanded Crenshaw's ideas.

In successive years, the concept of intersectionality has grown to include a broader range of disadvantage and oppression than feminism and race. Intersectionality is now a widely based concept that links together many inequalities, serving as a useful reminder for practitioners to acknowledge the different inequalities that can simultaneously affect an individual.

When you, as a professional, recognise a person's lack of confidence and diminished self-esteem, ask yourself whether intersectionality might be a causal factor. Indicating your awareness of intersectionality and then sensitively exploring the person's experiences of intersectionality when you communicate with them may help to overcome gaps in understanding. Sometimes a practitioner may be particularly interested in, and knowledgeable of, one aspect of intersectionality, such as racism. Another practitioner may be particularly interested in disability. The danger here is that discussion may become a competition between practitioners about which aspect is the most important for society to address. Every aspect of intersectionality is equally important, and many individuals' lives demonstrate the impact of several aspects: you may be communicating with an older disabled black woman, a bi-sexual asylum seeker or other individual who experiences combined aspects of intersectionality.

Practice example 2.1 A group of students nearing the end of their professional course had learned about several aspects of intersectionality, including but not limited to racism, sexism, and disablism. In discussion, a spirited argument developed about which 'ism' was the most devastating for an individual and therefore deserved the most attention and most generous government funding. The 'isms' became a competition during which the comparative severity of their impact was hotly debated. In response, their tutor reiterated the concept of the inter-woven nature of intersectionality and the futility of competing 'isms'.

A parallel debate sometimes takes place about the comparative value of the separate professions, their different purposes and styles of communication, and how the professions regard each other. This can sometimes lead to undervaluing the contributions of a particular profession within a team comprised of practitioners from different professions. A social worker may feel that their own contributions are not perceived with as high a regard as those of nurses. These feelings can impede communication and the quality of practice. A team that values each of its different professional team members and ensures open professional communication amongst its members is better enabled to deliver good practice.

First steps towards effective communication

Establishing effective communication is essential for professional practitioners. A 'good' communication is one that:

- is understood by the person who receives it
- conveys meaning accurately
- is offered with sensitivity and humanity

To enable professionals to practice effectively, the skills of communication are usually broken down into a phased process of separate steps.

The Shannon–Weaver model (1948, 1963) is a classic example of a stepped model of communication that was used widely in the 1960s and 1970s to help practitioners communicate effectively. This model describes concepts of the *sender or source of information* (the brain) that creates a message, selects a channel of communication, and transmits the message; the *encoder/transmitter* who sends the message using signals or binary data; the *channel*, which is the medium by which the message is sent; the *decoder* – the machine (or brain) that converts signals or binary data into a message; the *destination* (the place the message must reach) and the *receiver* (the person who gets the message). The *receiver* then provides feedback to the message. The Shannon–Weaver model uses the concept of *noise* to designate any interference that hinders the sending of the message – like radio static or a faulty TV signal. Shannon–Weaver identify three kinds of communication problems – technical, semantic (where the meaning of the message may be misunderstood by the receiver), and effectiveness, where the message may not evoke a desired reaction.

A simplified version of the model can be depicted through a diagram (Figure 2.1).

Although this model describes communication as a two-way process and recognises the importance of reducing the 'noise' that can hinder communication, in my view, the Shannon–Weaver model is mechanistic and impersonal, and fails to acknowledge the personal, social and psychological contexts of communication. It tries to create a scientific model of communication by breaking down the whole of communication into separate parts. Its merit lies in how it can help a practitioner plan the steps or phases of communication because it charts so clearly the sending of a communication, the receiving of a communication, and the range and types of 'noise' that get in the way of a clear reception of a communication.

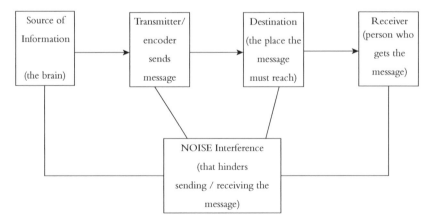

Figure 2.1 The Shannon–Weaver Model of Communication

Phases of communicating with a person

The next sections of this chapter discuss different phases of communication (introduction, assessment, engagement, and ending) and why it is important to recognise that social and psychological contexts shape people's lives and influence their communication.

Introductory phase: explaining role and purpose

The first step is to communicate with clarity: introduce yourself, your role, and the purpose of the communication. You need to be aware of how the other person perceives you, and identify possible barriers to communication.

> Practice example 2.2: A professional practitioner who speaks English with a different accent, introduces himself to a person who is requesting help for the first time. The person wonders about the practitioner's origins but is too shy to ask, and does not express her concern that the professional may not know enough English to be able to understand her. The person feels afraid. The practitioner could anticipate this reaction and reduce the person's anxiety by stating: 'You may have noticed that I speak English with a different accent. That is because I grew up in another country, but this country is my home now. Please let me know if you don't understand anything that I say or if I don't seem to understand what you say.' If the practitioner chooses this strategy, it is important to move on quickly from this revelation to the purpose of the conversation. This opening statement affirms the person's hidden thoughts, dispels worry, and conveys the message 'it's OK', but the practitioner should keep the focus on the person, rather than talk at length about themselves.

An introductory phase *provides* information (the role and identity of the practitioner, the reason for the contact, and its purpose) and also begins to *gather* information (asking questions of the person and observing interactions). After you gather this initial information, and take note of its content, you need to make sense of the communication, decide on the next steps, and communicate back what is likely to happen next.

The problem with these actions is that although you might adopt a logical approach, you may still fail to convey human engagement, empathy, and trust – human qualities that should be embedded within each step of the first communication, and then throughout the subsequent steps. Being human in your professional relationships demands sincerity, focus, and listening skills. Sometimes you may doubt your effectiveness, feel unsure, and worry that you are failing to communicate well. The person may be unresponsive, ill at ease, or hostile. Remember, the introductory phase means more than asking rote questions, it is a moment that is meant to 'set the scene' for communications that follow.

The anxious practitioner might consider him or herself to be unsuccessful in communicating with a service user if their dialogue is interrupted by children crying, a dog barking or a telephone ringing. If the communication takes place in an office setting, phone calls and staff entering the room may potentially threaten the flow of the communication. The Shannon–Weaver diagram indicates that 'noise' may interfere with a communication, but does not portray the often messy, interrupted dialogue that forms the communication.

Assessment phase

After the initial introduction, your communication will likely focus on getting to know the person, forming a relationship with them, gathering information about the person to determine whether and how your service can meet those particular needs – whether this is improvement in their health, psychological well-being, or seeking a different life style. As a practitioner, you are likely to follow certain steps when undertaking an assessment of needs, including using a designated pro-forma for your professional role.

Using a pro-forma can be alienating. If your concern is to complete the pro-forma as quickly and efficiently as possible, you will seem more interested in the mechanics of completing a form than in the person in front of you. The person may observe you becoming engrossed in your computer screen, not looking up, avoiding eye gaze, and firing questions in an impersonal manner. The person whose humanity is ignored during the assessment process is not likely to place his or her trust in you, or develop confidence in your professional ability. Here are some reminders for achieving a 'good' assessment:

- Look up, pause, and explain why you must ask certain questions.
- Explain what will happen to the information you obtain, and who will gain access to it.
- Encourage the person to ask questions about the process.
- Retain and share a sense of optimism about the end result of the assessment process.

You need to be clear whether the assessment is regarded as separate from, or part of, the helping process. In some organisations, an assessment pro-forma is completed by an employee who is not a professional practitioner, and then the form is handed over to the practitioner, who makes an appointment to see the client. In other organisations, the professional practitioner conducts an assessment that is incorporated into the helping process.

> *Practice example 2.3:* A social worker managed a small outreach centre in a rural community in the USA. She could choose to refer new clients with mental health needs to either of two mental health centres in the county town 25 miles away. After receiving her referrals, the first centre conducted an interview to assess the patient's needs, before assigning the patient to a professional practitioner for ongoing intervention. The second centre took a different approach, stating that 'intervention begins on day one'. Their staff conceptualised assessment as part of intervention, not separate from it. To them, the outreach social worker's initial contact with the patient was considered an intervention, and the assessment process was part of intervention.

> *Questions:* Which approach do you think was most successful in establishing good communication and a continuing commitment to seek help?
>   What are your reasons for your choice of approach?

The engagement phase: some essential considerations

The introductory phase has to win a person's trust, and this may take longer with some persons than with others. Individuals who seek help may be living lives burdened by fear, suspicion, and mistrust. Building trust is a necessary task for a practitioner. You can build trust by practising a *person-centred approach* developed by the psychologist Carl Rogers (1961), who argued that every individual has a potential for growth and development. Although Rogers published his method over fifty years ago, the *person-centred approach* remains popular and relevant. A professional practitioner who uses the person-centred approach will encourage the client's self-awareness and self-acceptance and will avoid being directive or authoritarian. Rogers stated that the person-centred approach requires six *necessary* and *sufficient* core conditions:

(1) The person and the professional practitioner are in contact with each other.
(2) The person is in a state of '*incongruence*', vulnerability or anxiety.
(3) The professional practitioner exhibits *congruence* in the relationship.
(4) The professional practitioner experiences *unconditional positive regard* towards the person.
(5) The professional practitioner experiences *empathetic understanding* of the person's internal frame of reference.
(6) The person perceives the professional practitioner's *unconditional positive regard* and empathetic understanding.

(Note that Rogers defined *congruence* as the *matching of experience and awareness*, and *incongruence* as *mismatching*.)

The six core conditions are sometimes condensed into three core conditions (empathy, unconditional positive regard, and genuineness.) Are these three conditions sufficient for bringing about change? Carkhuff's research findings maintained that the three conditions could bring about change '*for better or for worse*', depending on the skill of the professional (Carkhuff, 1984, p. 21). The person-centred approach is based on open, warm, accepting communication. When professional practitioners are distant in manner, they may seem overly mechanistic and technical. A practitioner's ability to communicate non-possessive warmth, concern, genuineness, empathy, non-judgemental acceptance, optimism and professional capability is likely to establish a positive therapeutic relationship. Not every practitioner agrees that Rogers' core conditions are 'sufficient' and instead may choose to combine elements of the person-centred approach with other approaches. The person-centred approach can function as a *binding force* that enables other approaches to come together to create a comprehensive strategy for helping. The counselling profession, the health professions, and the social work profession practise the person-centred approach. *Person-centred dementia care*, which developed from the observational research of Tom Kitwood and his associates (1997) views a person with dementia as an individual with *personhood*, arguing that person-centred care which emphasises social interactions can improve the individual's quality of life. Kitwood's linking of Rogers' theory to the care of individuals with dementia is a good example of how theoretical concepts can be brought together in practice.

Biestek's principles of the *casework relationship* (1992, 1957), written for social work practitioners, are similar to those of Rogers' person-centred approach. Although Rogers' ideas continue to exert an influence, particularly in counselling, Biestek's principles are less recognised within contemporary social work in the UK, probably because of increasing emphases on socio-legal interventions. Yet Biestek offers relevant ideas for communication. Biestek's principles include a non-judgemental attitude, practising with consistency and warmth, and offering acceptance. Accepting the person does not mean agreeing with all their actions and attitudes, but acknowledging our *shared humanity*.

Suggestions for practice

- Convey acceptance and trust with a look, a nod, or a restful pause, rather than by torrents of words.
- Remember that 'less is more': a few words can make a more positive impact than a flow of many words that may overwhelm the person.
- Convey reliability and consistency by turning up on time, or if you are unavoidably delayed, by informing the person that you will be late. By doing this, you show that you value the person and you value their reliability.

Active listening

Active listening (Rogers and Farson, 2015, 1957) requires alert attention to the person's verbal and non-verbal communication to help you understand the significance of that communication, and to respond appropriately and therapeutically. The practitioner should listen carefully but also observe the person's demeanour and be alert to possible obstacles that block the active listening process.

External obstacles include perceived differences in status between the practitioner and the person. Perceived power differentials of income, education, and verbal ability can impede attempts to build trust. Here we may recognise that the inequalities of inter-sectionality may sabotage a communication.

The ambience of the meeting venue can either enhance or detract from effective communication. Paying attention to ensuring a person's comfort will improve the com-munication (for example, by providing access to toilet facilities, a quiet room, commu-nicating in an audible volume, mediating any physical mobility difficulty, and enabling the person to understand and communicate through a mutually shared language).

Blocks to communication may arise – such as refusal or reluctance to accept suggestions, confusion, lack of empathy, incorrectly remembered data, erroneous assumptions, emo-tional distress, hard-to-understand language, missing non-verbal clues, being too distracted to listen properly, hidden personal prejudices, and unacknowledged negative attitudes. Again, intersectionality may underpin the client's feelings of being ill-at-ease. These psy-chological blocks may be triggered by the practitioner or by the person. Building trust will help you sustain the communication process. Through active listening and observation, you can identify possible obstacles to communication and take steps to overcome them. You may find that a person who has been required to accept professional help can feel coerced, and may become uncooperative. The professional practitioner needs to be aware of situations when this is the case, and take extra steps to build trust.

> Practice example 2.4: A university student contracted hepatitis and was hospitalised. After returning to the university (which was located in a rural area), the student felt depressed and was referred for therapy to an outpatient psychiatric clinic in a nearby city. She set her alarm early on the mornings of the weekly 9 a.m. appointment, walked a mile to the nearest bus route, and took two buses to arrive at the clinic on time. Each week the psychiatrist arrived 25 minutes late, and brushed past the student in the waiting room without saying anything. He never explained or apologised for his lateness. The student, awed by the psychiatrist's status and power, lacked the courage to comment on the lateness. She did not feel valued, and concluded that the psychiatrist would not be able to help her recover from her depression.

This example demonstrates that observed actions communicate effectively, in this instance, with a negative effect.

Question: How might this negative communication have been avoided?

Practice example 2.5: *A service user received regular visits from a social worker. Each time the social worker set an appointment for a specific time, but always arrived late, sometimes up to an hour beyond the appointment time. The social worker did not text or phone beforehand to inform the service user that she would be late, and when she arrived, did not apologise or explain. The service user was annoyed, but felt unable to express anger at the persistent lateness, because of the perceived power differential between the service user and the social worker. The service user felt unable to trust the social worker.*

The two different examples pose similar issues – whether the person can trust a professional practitioner when their relationship is damaged by persistent unexplained lateness, and whether unexplained lateness is unprofessional behaviour. Freud (1936, 2018) might interpret the behaviour as *transference* – a defence mechanism where the person perceives a practitioner's behaviour as being the same as behaviour from a previous relationship – and *counter-transference*, where without realising, a professional practitioner may transfer their reactions from a previous situation onto the present relationship.

Ending phase

There are two ways of looking at endings – first, when you end an interview or another kind of contact with a person, but you know you are likely to have ongoing contact with them. When ongoing contact is likely, drawing the communication to a close is relatively straightforward. You may say: 'it's time to stop now', and then arrange the next time you will meet or will be in touch. You may thank the person for sharing aspects of their situation with you, and summarise some positive aspects of the discussion – perhaps praising their courage in sharing a part of their life with you.

The second way of looking at endings is when the session is the last time you are likely to be in touch with the person. (Many professional services ration the number of contacts with the person.) When you come to the end of a final contact, you might spend time summarising what has been achieved together, and what might lie ahead for the person.

Practice example 2.6: *A woman in her late thirties who had experienced domestic violence and her children being taken into care, was reaching the end of six months of counselling with a charitable organisation. The counsellor used the last few sessions to write a short account of the woman's life story by consulting with her closely, and ensuring that the account emphasised the positive aspects of her life – her ability to plan, manage her money, and love her children – as well as the unhappy events of her life. At the last session, when the woman had agreed the contents, the counsellor gave her a copy of the life story to take with her.*

Our discussion so far has assumed that endings are always controlled by the professional, but sometimes, when contact is voluntary rather than statutorily required, the person may decide to end contact without explaining why. You may have thought that you were communicating well, or perhaps you noticed the person's reticence, anxiety, or annoyance. A key issue is how the person first made contact with you – did they come of their own accord or did a powerful entity in their life – a parent, a partner, or another professional practitioner – advise them to attend? Although they may present themselves as 'voluntary' they could feel that they were forced to see you. If this is so, they will have little motivation to continue and are likely to cease contact as soon as possible.

The significance of personal and social contexts for communication

Personal and social contexts are the environments in which each person lives – the house or flat, the neighbourhood, the people who are neighbours, friends, and family; and the employment, income, organisational attachments, leisure activities, health, choices of life style and the values and aspirations that give meaning to life. Personal and social contexts include the cultures and traditions that are part of people's identities. As well as here-and-now social contexts, each person is influenced by social contexts of their remembered past: life transitions, previous choices, moments of happiness and moments of loss.

Bronfenbrenner's *ecological systems theory* (1979) emphasised the importance of personal and social contexts, and his ideas are particularly relevant to human development, having led to the establishment of the child-focussed Head Start programmes in the USA and Sure Start programmes in the UK. Bronfenbrenner's ideas led to the creation of an ecological social work method for both children and adults (Teater, 2014; Germain and Gitterman, 1996), and to a method of ecological counselling (Cook, 2013). In the UK, Bronfenbrenner's theory is less recognised, but is nevertheless influential, and in my view, deserves to be better known. Bronfenbrenner conceptualised the *person-in-environment* interacting with four systems:

- the *micro-system* (intimate relationships, family relationships, social networks)
- the *meso-system* (relationships of individuals with institutions)
- the *exo-system* (the individual's relationships with distant organisations and institutions)
- the *macro-system* (cultural institutions of a society)

Personal and social contexts are an essential frame of reference for understanding a person. As you listen to a person's unfolding narratives, you will begin to recognise how personal and social contexts influence a person's dilemmas and life choices and become part of their perceptions of themselves and the world they live in. When engaged in person-to-person communication and interviewing, your awareness of a person's personal and social contexts will help you and the person to avoid stereotyped judgemental assumptions about the causes of problems.

> Practice example 2.7: An older woman reported experiencing feelings of guilt and depression. She worried about the cost of electricity, so she checked the electricity meter every day. This had become a ritual, influenced by her memory of her late mother being very worried about the cost of electricity. The woman was not able to acknowledge that she herself had a good retirement income, owned a

car, and had ample savings. Her fear about electricity bills derived from her memory of her mother's social context and her own mistaken guilt that she had not done enough for her mother.

This account of how personal and social contexts from the past influence present behaviours also acknowledges that psychological contexts are important influences. By using empathetic supportive communication, a professional practitioner could help the woman recognise how personal and social contexts from the past were influencing her present psychological contexts and were diminishing her emotional well-being.

Summarising the chapter: the theme of shared humanity

Valuing a person so that you can communicate effectively requires recognition of *shared humanity*. As human beings, we are distinct individuals with different personalities, abilities, and appearances, and we share the struggle of trying to balance intellectual convictions and emotional feelings. We recognise that we have flaws, but sometimes deny them; we sometimes feel pity and compassion towards others, but also anger and hostility. These contradictions typify what it is to be a human being. Shared humanity can build a bridge of understanding between human differences and reach out across the divide of the many aspects of intersectionality. Humanity enables us to recognise the precious quality of individuality and the vulnerability of human life, and so, to be effective, communication must take note of shared humanity.

References

Beresford, P. (2016) *All Our Welfare: Towards Participatory Social Policy*. Policy Press: London.

Beresford, Peter (2012) 'What service users want from social workers' *Community Care*, 27 April 2012,http://www.communitycare.co.uk/2012/04/27/what-service-users-want-from-social-workers/ website accessed 10 June 2018.

Beresford, P. (2009) *Compass think piece 47: whose personalisation?* Compass: London.

Beresford, P. (2000) 'Service Users' Knowledges and Social Work Theory: Conflict or Collaboration?' *British Journal of Social Work*, Volume 30, Issue 4, pp. 489–504.

Biestek, F. (1992, 1957) *The Casework Relationship*. Routledge: London.

Bronfenbrenner, U. (1979) *The Ecology of Human Development*. Harvard University Press: Cambridge, MA.

Carkhuff, R.R. (1984, 1969) *Helping and Human Relations* (2 volumes). Human Resource Development Press: Amherst, MA.

Collins, Patricia Hill (2000, 1990) *Black Feminist Thought: Knowledge, Consciousness and the Politics of Empowerment* (Perspectives on Gender). Routledge: New York.

Collins, Patricia Hill, and Bilge, Sirma (2016) *Intersectionality*. Polity Press: Cambridge.

Cook, Ellen P. (2013) *Understanding People in Context: The Ecological Perspective in Counselling*. American Counselling Association. Wiley: Hoboken NJ.

Crenshaw, K. (1989) 'Demarginalizing the Intersection of Race and Sex: A Black Feminist Critique of Antidiscrimination Doctrine, Feminist Theory and Anti Racist Politics'. The University of Chicago Legal Forum. 140: 139–167.

Freud, A. (2018, 1936) *The Ego and the Mechanisms of Defense*. Routledge: Abingdon.

Germain, C.D. and Gitterman, A. (1996) *The Life Model of Social Work Practice*. 2nd Edition. Columbia University Press: New York.

Kitwood, T. (1997) *Dementia Reconsidered. The Person Comes First.* Open University Press: Buckingham.

Rogers, C. R. (1961) *On Becoming a Person* Constable: London.

Rogers, Carl, and Farson, Richard (2015, 1957) *Active Listening.* Martino Fine Books: Mansfield Center, CT: (originally published by the Industrial Relations Center, University of Chicago: Chicago).

Shannon, Claude Elwood and Weaver, Warren (1963, 1948) 'The Mathematical Theory of Communication', *Bell System Technical Journal*, University of Illinois Press: Chicago.

Teater, B. (2014) 'Social work practice from an ecological perspective' in C.W. Lecroy (ed.) *Case Studies in Social Work Practice*. 3rd Edition. Brooks Cole: Belmont, CA.

Chapter 3

The professional practitioner

Personal and social contexts and the public's changing perceptions of different helping professions

Persons who receive services live within different personal and social contexts (discussed in Chapter 2) that influence their perception of self. The mass media and internet have created shared personal and social contexts for us all. Our shared contexts are more open than in previous years, information is easily available, and people feel more able to question practitioners and to query the services they receive. Media revelations of inequalities and injustices in public services have increased public doubt about the trustworthiness of professional standards. As a result, deference to authority is no longer as dominant a feature of our modern society as it once was.

Members of the public perceive different helping professions in different ways, and their perceptions affect how they communicate with professional practitioners. The public may perceive that health services are on the brink of collapse, and could damage people's health rather than curing them; they read about social workers taking children away from their parents and putting older people into homes without regard for individual rights; they may think of counselling as mysterious and frightening. This is not a wholly accurate picture, of course; the public does hear about practitioners' positive achievements, but doubt and disillusionment have chipped away at public trust. Consequently, a practitioner may find that a person's anxiety, reticence, fear and/or hostility impede attempts to communicate.

Considerable patience, insight, and skill are needed to overcome these barriers. A key issue is whether a practitioner is perceived as trustworthy. Because the class structure has weakened in British society, deferential responses to people who used to be perceived as one's 'betters' can no longer be assumed. Practitioners' authority is cast into doubt. For an individual practitioner, there is no easy remedy for this, but if practitioners communicate clearly, openly, and honestly, and explain issues clearly, they will begin to build trust. If they speak in jargon, seem not to listen, and fail to explain difficult issues clearly, they will appear to communicate an absence of humanity and convey a probable use of covert power. Suspicion and fear will set up an emotional barrier to building trust.

Professional practitioners work in 'people services' – social work, counselling, health professions and other services like youth services – where styles of communication are likely to vary. The health professions have traditionally assumed a more authoritarian manner than other professions. Dealing with the impact of disease and injuries led historically to a disciplined authoritarian approach to fight infection. Unsanitary living conditions and the absence of antibiotics made this necessary, but this approach has changed, and is now likely to include an educational element of sharing information and providing explanations to the patient. Practitioners may need to remind themselves that the decreasing prominence of an overt authoritarian manner in the professions cannot entirely remove the fear of power and control that clients/patients/users of services can feel, but not be able to express.

Similarities and differences in professional approaches

Similarities and differences in helping roles sometimes create a gulf between professionals, or alternatively, enable beneficial sharing of ideas and approaches. Professional practitioners are likely to develop different communication styles depending on their professional roles and the purpose of their communications. Practitioners' awareness of their clients/patients/service users' personal and social contexts, and of the impact of *intersectionality* on their lives will help them modify certain communication styles in favour of more open exchanges of information.

Health professions

Physicians in general practice typically diagnose and treat the patient within a limited time frame of about 10 minutes. They are obliged to communicate within a short time frame, at the same time establishing and maintaining trust. Nurses and other health practitioners (for example, occupational therapists and physiotherapists) communicate with their patients for varying lengths of time, depending on the purpose of the intervention.

> Practice example 3.1 In a busy medical practice with six general practitioners, signs were placed on the GP office doors stating: 'Your appointment is for 10 minutes only and you may raise one topic only.' Some patients objected to the preemptory tone of these signs, and felt less valued as a consequence, even though they acknowledged the time pressures on the doctors.
>
> *Question:* What might have been a better way of communicating this message?

Paternalistic models of communication

Physicians have traditionally used a paternalistic model of communication, based on their own autonomy and self-determination (Wilson–Barnett, 1986, 1989; Childress, 1982) as well as the assumption of authority and responses of public deference. The paternalistic practitioner initiates a communication and directs it towards the person. The paternalistic model is authoritarian and expects patient compliance and gratitude in return.

> Practice example 3.2 Patients in a busy GP practice that employed several doctors commented that one of the doctors was less popular than the others. The doctor was clinically accurate and reliable, but patients perceived him as authoritarian, and demonstrating little human

concern. He showed no emotions in his gaze and facial expressions, spoke in a flat authoritarian tone, and did not welcome questions.

A different approach to health care now challenges this paternalistic model. The doctor/
patient relationship is no longer the only significant health care relationship. The patient is
now likely to form relationships with other members of the health care team – nurses,
physiotherapists, health care assistants. In England, general practitioners are encouraged to
join group practices rather than work as single practitioners. The general practitioner team
confers with each other over patient care, thus increasing the different layers of communication. The patient may make appointments to see other general practitioners in the
practice, rather than their own named GP, particularly if this means securing an earlier
appointment. The doctor/patient relationship now takes place within a network of other
professional relationships that have the capacity to increase the quality of patient care, but
which may also become more impersonal.

Practice example 3.3 A male patient with high blood pressure met with the practice nurse
twice a year, saw the phlebotomist twice when blood samples were drawn for testing, and
interacted with many of the practice staff when the staff delivered mass inoculations against
winter influenza. He felt well cared for by the practice team, but did not have a personal
relationship with his GP or any other staff member. He did not visit his GP at any other point
in the year because his health issues were dealt with satisfactorily by the practice staff.

Participatory model

Traditional power structures are being modified in favour of communication which resembles
a *participatory development communication* model that was developed to empower community
development projects (Tufte and Mefalopulos, 2009). Communication in general practice is
now a multi-layered process, with physicians communicating with patients and health staff in
more open ways. This more open style of communication requires health practitioners to
establish mutually acceptable levels of communication for expressing and resolving different
opinions about what is best for a patient, and for raising issues of poor practice.

The *paternalistic model* of communication does not fit easily with the *participatory model*,
in which the doctor (or other health practitioner) and the patient participate together in
exchanging information, responding and asking questions. Challenges to the *paternalistic
model* of health care coincided with the trial and conviction of Dr. Harold Shipman, a
general practitioner who murdered over 200 of his older patients without detection over
a number of years. Subsequently, the Shipman Inquiry Fifth Report (2004) recommended more checks and balances to modify the traditional health care power structure.
Doctors now have to be licensed and certificated in order to practice, be appraised
annually, and be revalidated (involving re-licensing and re-certification) every five years.

The patient's trust may no longer be given automatically, but must be earned. Care
partnerships that communicate informatively with patients are more prevalent. Internet
access enables patients to research their symptoms and illnesses. Patient groups, self-help
groups, and complaints systems provide more voices and power to patients, thus strength-
ening the argument that the predominant model of communication is now *participatory*.

Constructivist model

Professional practitioners and persons who receive services may find it helpful to adopt a *constructivist model* of communication to mitigate moments of delivering or receiving disappointing news. A *constructivist model* is a theory of creative learning, in which persons draw on their previous knowledge and experience to evaluate new experiences and then construct a new kind of understanding (Piaget, 1971; Wadsworth, 2004). We might think of the constructivist model as 'making the best of things' – a strategy for remaining hopeful when faced with difficult dilemmas. Victor Frankl might call this strategy a *search for meaning* (2014; 2011, 1969). Frankl's emphasis on this search for meaning needs to be understood in the context of his survival of World War II concentration camps. In a constructivist model of communication, the person who is at the receiving end of service provision finds their own particular meaning in a situation and exercises their own power to understand and respond to their situation, rather than defer to authority. The *constructivist model* is compatible with concepts of personal and social contexts and *intersectionality* as influences on communication.

> Practice example 3.4 A man in his fifties experienced pain in his eyes, but did not consider the pain significant until being diagnosed with a detached retina. Following a complex operation, his eyesight was saved, but left him impaired with double vision. He researched his condition fully on the internet, because he wanted to know everything about his condition. He visited his GP, who spoke to him sympathetically and commented that he could perhaps consider himself fortunate, because in previous years he would been completely blind. The man appreciated the doctor's constructive way of looking at his situation.

Next, the man visited his optician for new spectacles.

> Practice example 3.5: The optician examined his eyes, and explained the complexities of his eye condition, how spectacles might help to improve his vision, but told him that he would never be able to drive again. The man said he appreciated her knowledge, honesty, and sympathetic manner. He liked receiving full information, being able to ask questions, and being treated with respect. He felt better equipped to face the future despite knowing that he could never go back to his old job. He commented that he and his wife felt fortunate that their mortgage was paid off and they had no debts, thus adopting a constructivist frame of mind to sustain his recovery.

This example shows a patient responding positively to the full information he was given. He respected rather than feared the power of professional practitioners because he felt they kept him fully informed. He was ready to face his situation because of his experience of informative, trustworthy professional practitioners.

The social model and the medical model

Social work's professional qualifying courses frequently teach the *social model* that promotes service user participation to change the way services are organised. They criticise the *medical model*, where professional power is said to be paramount, looking at what is 'wrong' with a person and not what a person needs. Oliver (1983, 1989, 1996) developed these as two contrasting models of disability, but the models are now often discussed as referring to all health and social services. Regrettably, this social work teaching has negatively influenced social workers' perceptions of health practitioners and hindered inter-professional communication. Social workers hopefully will acknowledge changes in health care that seek to move practice away from an authoritarian paternalistic *medical model* towards a more *participatory social model*.

Social workers

Social workers try to practice the *participatory model* of communication, based on their informal partnerships with service user groups and complaints systems. Social workers usually work within a social work team and communicate with persons who use services for short or long periods of time, depending on the purpose of the contact. Social workers may be required to use lengthy assessment pro-formas with persons who use services and to discuss statutory and legal requirements while also trying to establish trust. Social workers' engagement with legal frameworks and safeguarding requirements tend to evoke an authoritarian model of practice. In some areas, the social workers may be members of health and social work multi-professional teams, but that is not the current dominant organisational model. Social workers in mental health teams and hospitals are more likely to communicate on a regular basis with health service practitioners.

Social workers practise in pressured circumstances, and although they receive line management supervision, do not always, at the present time, receive professional reflective supervision which would allow them to explore their practice dilemmas and the impacts of the stressful situations they encounter on their well-being. In conversation they sometimes perceive themselves to be underappreciated and misunderstood – hence they sometimes assert informally '*we are the social model and health is the medical model*'. Social workers sometimes express frustration about their public image, knowing that the tabloid press is quick to heap blame on social work actions. Although they practise a wide range of skills, they may feel hard pressed to identify a particular area of knowledge and skill that is distinctive to social work. My view is that social workers' knowledge and understanding of service users' personal and social contexts and *intersectionality* is distinctive and should be more widely recognised.

Counsellors

Counsellors generally practise individually, seeing their clients alone and not practising as part of a team. Counselling time frames differ from those of health care: the counsellor typically has 50 minutes to interact with the client, build and sustain trust, and select appropriate techniques for addressing the identified issues. Counsellors now practise in the health service to deliver cognitive behavioural therapy (CBT) and other therapies through the IAPT (Improved Access to Psychological Therapies) programme, where they usually work on a one-to-one basis. Their isolation poses risks that counsellors may unwittingly slip into a *paternalistic model* in relation to the client. Counsellors must adhere to a professional requirement to practise according to an ethical code and to meet monthly with a professional supervisor. It is less clear at the current time how counselling clients' collective voices can raise concerns about counselling practice. Counsellors do not have a protected title and are regulated through voluntary registers rather than a statutory register. One might question whether counselling is moving towards a *participatory model* of communication or whether its mode of communication is in fact, more authoritarian than is currently recognised.

Therapeutic relationships

Social work's therapeutic, relationship-based *social model* of intervention, which Hood (2018) argues has lost ground to managerial legalistic models of practice, is indebted to Rogers' person-centred approach (1961). This means that communication with persons who use services traditionally takes place within the context of a *therapeutic relationship*. Therapeutic relationships also are important in health care and counselling. Biestek (1992, 1957) and Rogers (1961) both argued for the importance of *relationships* in practice, a concept that emerged from attempts to identify the essence of a helping interaction in terms of personal qualities rather than precise skills. Perlman, a pioneering American social work academic, historically promoted the importance of relationships (1983, 1979) in therapeutic interventions, arguing that the quality of the therapeutic relationship between the professional and the person was a large factor in achieving positive outcomes. Perlman (ibid., p. 71) urged the therapist to demonstrate that he or she is 'at one' with the person – feeling not *like* the person, but *with* the person. A therapeutic relationship – characterised by empathetic understanding, rapport, openness, and trust between the person and the professional, so that both work together to attain agreed outcomes – is the opposite of a *paternalistic* or '*medical*' model of practice. Nevertheless, in today's world, it tends to be counselling rather than social work that emphasises the importance of relationships.

Rapport and empathy

Rapport (Egan, 2013, 1985) – a close, harmonious relationship – and *empathy* (Egan, 2013, 1985) – the ability to understand and share another's feelings – are two frequently mentioned qualities of a therapeutic relationship. Both qualities are importanant for professional practice (Workman, 2013). *Rapport* links practice to a particular values stance and communication style. Building *rapport* resembles Shulman's description of 'tuning in' (1984, in Devore and Schlesinger, 1991, pp. 196–198), which describes how the professional practitioner develops preparatory *empathy* through attempts to get in touch with feelings that are either implicitly or explicitly expressed. Practitioners can observe the interwoven, related nature of the practice theories.

Empathy is a related concept that sometimes is considered the same as *rapport*. *Empathetic responding* involves understanding what the person is saying from an internal personal frame of reference, reflecting on the content, and the feelings that are expressed, and then communicating back your understanding in language the person can understand (Nelson-Jones, 2014, 1983, pp. 40–64). Despite a longstanding value given to the quality of empathy, Bloom (2016) has adopted a more critical stance, arguing that empathy is never sufficient on its own as a single helping approach, and that *rational compassion* should be substituted for *empathy*. Empathy is solely the heart/soul/emotion of helping; rational compassion combines the *heart* with the *head/reason/thinking approach*.

The assumption that *rapport, empathy,* and *relationship* are therapeutic tools for good communication has suffered something of an eclipse in popularity as the *evidence-based practice* movement (Marsh and Fisher, 2005) gained prominence. Advocates of evidence-based practice sought to make practice more like a 'science' than an 'art' (Keith-Lucas, 1972), but I suggest that professional communication benefits from the 'art' as well as the 'science' of practice and should include therapeutic relationships, *rapport,* and *empathy.* The challenge to practitioners is how they can manage to balance the 'science' of practice, often embodied by the need to implement socio-legal procedures, with the 'art' of practice, characterised by human responses of empathy, listening, and compassion. The issue of clients' lack of trust (discussed earlier in the chapter), which is prompted by fear of the power of the professional practitioner, can be a sabotaging factor in the practitioner's desire to respond with empathy.

Differences in cultural and ethnic identities

Establishing *rapport* between a practitioner and the person may pose a challenge when cultural and ethnic identities differ. As well as experiencing a lack of trust and fearing the power of the professional practitioner, the person seeking help may feel that someone from a different cultural and ethnic identity will not understand or be sympathetic to their situations. Ramirez (1999) advises that when engaging with persons from an ethnic identity different from one's own, a professional practitioner should develop 'cultural flex' (flexibility of approach) to take these differences into account. Being able to view the world through the eyes of a person whose ethnic and cultural background differs from the practitioner's own identity requires *empathetic projection* to achieve a state of rapport. Ramirez recommends starting with friends or family members whose values may differ from your own, or reading autobiographies of people with different identities and values.

Some suggested protocols for communicating with a person who seeks help from you

Your use of language

- Speak **slowly** and clearly throughout – do not 'gabble'!
- Use **plain English**
- Avoid **jargon**
- Avoid **colloquialisms** and **stereotyped cultural assumptions**
- Avoid professional **acronyms**
- If the person does not understand English, and you cannot speak their language, arrange for an **interpreter**
- Ensure that the person(s) can **hear you**

Essential information for you to share

- Introduce yourself by your **name** and **professional role**
- Introduce any **others** who may be present and their **roles**.

- Explain **why** they are present
- Explain the **purpose** of the meeting
- Inform the person(s) of your organisation's **complaints/appeal** process

Communication techniques

- Invite the person's **comments** and ask for their **views**
- Use **open-ended** questions
- Ensure that your communication has been **understood**
- Encourage **questions** from the person who uses services
- Clarify the **information** that you communicate to the person
- Explain the scope and limits of **confidentiality**, and what will happen to the information that is shared
- Do not refer to **legislation or policies** without explaining their meaning
- Don't be afraid to say **'I don't know'**; you can find the relevant information later
- **Recapitulate** and **summarise** the content of your discussion

These bullet points may seem daunting, but over time and with ongoing efforts to practice these skills, you will be able to use this communication protocol with confidence and ease.

Practice example 3.7 A woman (who was subjected to an investigation by social services to find out whether her young child was experiencing significant harm) was required to attend meetings convened by social services where twelve professional practitioners were present. The mother said afterwards that she could not remember what was said, the discussion was a blur, and the chairperson used many professional abbreviations without explaining them. The woman was unable to comprehend what was being said, and she did not know the name of the chairperson.

Question: How would you improve the communication at the meeting?

Summary

Your own style of communication is an individual activity that draws on the essence of your 'self' in a uniquely personal way but nevertheless will be based on the ethics of your profession. The art of practice (Samson, 2015; Keith-Lucas, 1972) is to learn how to communicate effectively and appropriately in your professional role. Communication is a skill that is acquired, enhanced, and understood through practice, learning, and reflection over time. Experienced practitioners usually learn the basic principles of communication in their first year of training and education, but may find that they drift away from these principles particularly when they are fatigued or stressed.

Despite differences in professional roles, core elements of good communication practice are shared across the professions. Communicating with the person who receives services, or who is a client or a patient, means entering into the world of the person – their personal contexts and taking note of the social contexts that shape their world, as well as aspects of *intersectionality*.

> - You can achieve good communication by establishing rapport and empathy, using Rogers' person-centred approach (1961).

Active listening and being attentive to the person are essential skills.

> - Invite the person to tell his or her story or concerns – ask 'how are you doing?' or 'how have things been for you?'
> - Try to avoid asking too many direct questions.

Remember, as you listen and respond, that your communication is a creative shared process.

> - Be yourself, and develop your own style, whilst observing the principles and ethics of good communication.

References

Biestek, F. (1992, 1957) *The Casework Relationship*. Routledge: London.

Bloom, P. (2016) *Against Empathy: The Case for Rational Compassion*. Ecco Press: Harper Collins: New York.

Childress, James F. (1982) *Who Should Decide? Paternalism in Health Care*. Oxford University Press: London.

Devore, W. and Schlesinger, E. G. (1991) *Ethnic-Sensitive Social Work Third Edition*. Merrill, Macmillan: New York.

Egan, G. (1985) *The Skilled Helper: A Systematic Approach to Effective Helping*. Brooks/Cole Publishing: Belmont, CA.

Egan, G. (2013) *The Skilled Helper: A Problem Management and Opportunity Development Approach to Helping*. Brooks/Cole Publishing: Belmont, CA.

Frankl, V. (2014) *The Will to Meaning: Foundations and Applications of Logotherapy*. Meridian: London.

Frankl, V. (2011, 1969) *Man's Search for Ultimate Meaning*. Basic Books: Cambridge, MA.

Hood, Rick (2018) *Complexity in Social Work*. Sage: London.

Keith-Lucas, A. (1972) *Giving and Taking Help*. University of North Carolina Press: Chapel Hill, N.C.

Keith-Lucas, A. (1972) 'The Art and Science of Helping' in Timms, N. and Watson, D. (eds) (1976) *Talking about Welfare: Readings in Philosophy and Social Policy*, Library Editions: Welfare and the State. Routledge and Kegan Paul: Henley

Marsh, Peter, and Fisher, Mike (2005) *Developing the Evidence Base for Social Work and Social Care*. Social Care Institute for Excellence: London.

Nelson-Jones, R. (2014, 1983) *Practical Counselling and Helping Skills Sixth Edition*. Sage: London.

Oliver, M. (1983) *Social Work with Disabled People*. Macmillan: Basingstoke.

Oliver, M. (1989) 'The social model of disability: current reflections' in Carter, P.Jeffs, T. and Smith, M. (eds.) *Social Work and Social Welfare Yearbook I*, Open University: Milton Keynes, pp. 190–203.

Oliver, M. (1996) *Understanding Disability: From Theory to Practice*. Macmillan: Basingstoke.

Perlman, H. H. (1971, 1957) *Social Casework: A Problem Solving Process*. University of Chicago Press: Chicago.

Perlman, H. H. (1983, 1979) *Relationship: The Heart of Helping People*. University of Chicago Press: Chicago.

Piaget, J. (1971). 'The theory of stages in cognitive development' in Green, D. R., Ford, M. P. and Flamer, G. B., *Measurement and Piaget*. McGraw-Hill: New York.

Ramirez, M. (1999, 1991) *Psychotherapy and Counseling with Minorities. A Cognitive Approach to Individual and Cultural Differences*. Pergamon Press: New York.

Rogers, C. R. (1961) *On Becoming a Person*. Constable: London.

Samson, P. (2015) Practice Wisdom: The Art and Science of Social Work. *Journal of Social Work Practice*, Volume 29, Issue 2, pp. 119–131.

Shipman Inquiry Fifth Report (2004) *Safeguarding Patients: Lessons from the Past – Proposals for the Future*. National Archives http://webarchive.nationalarchives.gov.uk/20090808155110/http://www.the-shipman-inquiry.org.uk/reports.asp. Website accessed 6 June 2019.

Shulman, L. (1984) *The Skills of Helping: Individuals and Groups* 2nd Edition. F.E. Peacock: Itasca, Illinois.

Tufte, T. and Mefalopulos, P. (2009) Participatory Communication: a practical guide. World Bank Working Paper; no 170 World Bank: Washington DC.

Wilson-Barnett, Jenifer (1989) 'Limited autonomy and partnership: professional relationships in health care', *Journal of Medical Ethics*, Volume 15, pp. 12–16.

Wilson-Barnett, Jenifer (1986) 'Ethical Dilemmas in Nursing', *Journal of Medical Ethics, Volume* 12, Issue 30, pp. 123–135.

Wadsworth, B. J. (2004). *Piaget's theory of cognitive and affective development: Foundations of constructivism*. Longman Publishing: London.

Workman, Stephen R. (2013) 'The Importance of Establishing a Rapport with Patients' *British Medical Journal*, Volume 347, published 25 September 2013.

Chapter 4

Different communication approaches: essential tools of practice

This chapter explains how patient/service user/client groups have changed the nature of professional communication, resulting in practitioners listening to the views of people who use services. The *heart/soul/emotions* approach to communication is contrasted with the *head/mind/reason* approach. The chapter explores the *heart/soul/emotion* aspect of practice though some classic texts that have been developed further by contemporary researchers:

- use of *relationships* (Biestek,1992, 1957)
- *use of self* (Dewane, 2006) and the
- *art of practice* (England, 1986)

Choosing different communication approaches

Choosing appropriate communication approaches helps practitioners and people who use services achieve agreed aims. Approaches should be compatible with theoretical approaches and personal styles, and fit with the purpose of employer organisations. Alternatively, some attempts at communication may be disastrous exchanges that fail to achieve their purposes. Personal preferences, professional roles, and the purpose of a particular communication influence a practitioner's choice of approach. The skilled practitioner selects a communication approach in a flexible manner, and recognises the importance of careful listening and retaining an open mind.

> *Practice example 4.1: A class of young professional students voiced objections to presenting themselves differently when working as a professional practitioner. They claimed that wearing formal clothing (a jacket and tie, a tailored dress or trouser suit), for a job interview or a court hearing, and using a formal vocabulary was false, because that was not how they usually presented themselves. Their attitude was 'I am who I am — take it or leave it'. Perhaps they felt insecure about their adult sense of self. The suggestion that versatility is a good communication trait was threatening to them at that stage of their professional development, but as their experience and confidence grew, they learned to expand their repertoire of communication and become more flexible in their approach.*

A repertoire of communication

Your repertoire of communication as a professional practitioner will include both informal and formal modes of conversation.

- Informal modes (verbal and non-verbal communication, including telephone conversations) help to establish relationships, express human concern, and convey hope, or alternatively express anger, fear, and doubt.
- Formal modes (written communication, email, Skype, meetings, and texts) inform, convey a precise message, argue a point, or make formal presentations.

> Sometimes the lines between formal and informal communications get blurred.
> *Question:* What are the key features of these different modes of communication?

Informal modes of communication

Verbal communication

Verbal communications are used often for informal messages – laughter, shared reminiscences, information about family and friends, as well as formal exchanges of thoughts and opinions. Confrontations, anger, and tears are verbal communications that convey negative emotions. Formal meetings depend on verbal communication (as well as written reports), but these words later become part of a written record of proceedings.

Verbal messages can establish a relationship, convey concern and understanding, and offer support. Some examples of verbal communication that build relationships include:

> - *How are you today?* (Invite the person to tell their story)
> - *That must have been a concern/worrying/upsetting for you.* (Share concern, recognise the person's feelings and worries)
> - *Last week you mentioned that…* (Communicate that you remember something of what has been happening)

Non-verbal communication

Non-verbal communication conveys messages through body posture, gestures, and facial expressions.

> - A person who feels tense and anxious may unwittingly adopt a worried expression or an angry look, and sit awkwardly.
> - Avoiding eye gaze suggests that the person may be afraid of sharing something important.
> - A frown may indicate worry.
> - A smile may indicate trust and relief, or alternatively embarrassment or disbelief.

The professional practitioner will realise that these interpretations are guesswork until they can be verified by verbal communication.

- Non-verbal communication provides hints of the person's emotional state and should not be ignored.
- A few words of encouragement may release verbal communication about inner feelings, but if the person chooses not to reveal themself, that decision must be respected.

Sometimes a professional practitioner may unknowingly use inappropriate non-verbal communication.

Practice example 4.2 A prospective client met with a counsellor for an initial assessment. The client spoke openly about their past life, including the death of a sister. The counsellor wrote down the information without comment, but grimaced in response to the information about the sister's death. The facial grimace communicated apparent shock and negative emotion. The prospective client said nothing at the time, but later pondered this facial expression and found it disturbing. Consequently the client decided not to return and cancelled the next appointment.

Was the counsellor aware of this involuntary facial expression? Perhaps the counsellor revealed a spontaneous emotional reaction that, when viewed by the client, seemed incompatible with professional respect. The client concluded that the counsellor was either upset by the revelation, or disapproving, or perhaps unable to deal with the issue effectively.

Informal ways of establishing a relationship

In traditional British culture, offering and accepting a cup of tea (or coffee) can be a positive social gesture to welcome a person and help them feel more at ease. The practitioner may offer a cup of tea to the person, or the person may offer one to the practitioner who visits the person's home. Not everyone, however, wants a cup of tea. Declining the offer is acceptable if done politely. Sometimes offering or accepting a glass of water is an acceptable alternative.

Referring to sporting events and popular culture may help to form a relationship, but may become divisive, if the person is not interested in or knowledgeable of those topics. In a mixed gender group, some popular topics may help the practitioner make a connection with male participants, and other topics may strike a chord with the women, but the practitioner risks favouring some participants over others, or being too gender-specific, or making assumptions about a person's interests, and possibly excluding some persons from full understanding.

The use of humour can sometimes help to form a relationship, but also can be a pitfall. The listener may not understand some jokes or may perceive them as offensive because of the language used. The use of humour often assumes a shared culture between the teller of the joke and the listener, but a shared culture of beliefs and perceptions may not actually exist. A better strategy is to first try to become acquainted with the person's culture and interests before assuming that certain interests are shared and known universally.

Practice Example 4.3 A woman visited her GP, and described her feelings of desperation, saying that these were prompted by her husband's recent behaviour. The GP responded with the comment 'he bowled you a googly there'. The woman looked blank and mystified, not understanding the cricket term which means to bowl an off-spin ball with a leg-break action, i.e. deliberately deceiving the batsman.

Formal modes of communication

Books, articles, and reports

Books, articles, and reports may appear to have an air of finality about them, but the astute reader will scrutinise the evidence that backs up the arguments in the document, and examine the language used. Consider the date when a book or article was published: does its message remain relevant to today's social contexts? Did the book introduce new ideas? Did it become a classic text? Not all newly published material is of the same standard, and part of the professional role is to be able to discern the quality of a written communication. Older texts need to be evaluated in terms of their influence on current practice and their ability to generate new ideas and approaches for practice.

- Does the language try so hard to capture your allegiance that it loses credibility?
- A non-fiction book or article should be carefully referenced; but some publications contain many references and are so cautious in tone that they may slow down the reader's comprehension.

Formal communication should use plain English. The Plain English Campaign has campaigned since 1979 against 'gobbledygook, jargon and misleading public information' (http://www.plainenglish.co.uk, accessed 10 June 2018) and believes that every person should be able to access clear information. To help the public, their website contains, for example, guides on design and layout, advice on how to use financial, legal, and pension terms, and medical information.

Practitioners should avoid using

- an overly academic style that communicates mainly to other people in academic roles
- a very informal style that communicates only with 'in-groups'
- acronyms and jargon that are not widely known to the general public

Practitioners demonstrate good formal communication when they create coherent written structures that contain accurate information in a format with

- an introduction
- paragraphs

- sub-headings
- a conclusion that summarises key points
- a glossary of technical terms, and
- accurate references

Reports, formal letters, committee minutes and agendas, and practice records, may be extracted and used for court hearings at a later date, so it is important to proofread carefully and aim for accuracy. Email messages and text messages circulate widely, but are they seen as informal or formal communication? I suggest that any information that is written down and circulates widely should be treated as formal communication that must be checked for accuracy and impact before circulation.

How do persons acquire information?

We read and learn from media-based information and from formal written communications from official organisations, but we may have difficulty understanding written communication that contains many *technical terms, jargon and acronyms*. Some persons may have difficulty distinguishing accurate information from false information. (Chapter 7 discusses 'information giving' as a means of building individual confidence and helping people decide on what actions to take.)

Practice example 4.5 A student tentatively asked her lecturer 'Is everything in the newspapers and social media true?' The student was accustomed to gaining knowledge from tabloid newspapers and social media, and she believed everything she read. Then doubts began to creep in. She began to realise that there might be alternative explanations of events. Her lecturer praised the student's growing discernment and suggested that she continue to evaluate the accuracy of media information.

Communicating via emails, text messages, and social media

Increasing numbers of people now communicate via emails, text messages, and social media groups. Sometimes these communications can be misunderstood if individual exchanges of communication take place quickly without accompanying non-verbal communication. In a group social media context, miscommunication can have wide-ranging ramifications, often negative and unwittingly destructive. The professional practitioner needs to be aware of the unintended consequences of using these methods of communication, particularly the dangers of blurring professional and personal information, and of communicating potentially harmful inferences.

Technology can offer learning opportunities to new audiences via online courses. Yet there is a danger that learning will become impersonal and overly formal in style, robbing the learner of opportunities to communicate with a tutor and other learners. Jonasson et al. (1995, 2009) advocate adopting a constructive participative communication approach to using computer technology for learning purposes, so that educators avoid allowing the technology to unwittingly lead them to deliver a one-way authoritarian lecture to passive learners. Instead, educators are urged to use the technology to set up collaborative feedback and discussions, so the learning is a two-way endeavour that enables learners to communicate with each other and with the educator. Used in this way, the technology can facilitate a search for meaning and reflection on practice.

Group communication skills

Group communication skills are important for professional practitioners who regularly attend staff/practice meetings, conferences, multi-professional meetings, and reviews. Some practitioners at first may find it difficult to participate, perhaps because of inexperience and/or fear of appearing foolish in front of others who seem more expert. To get started, you might gain confidence by

- Stating your appreciation of a colleague's contribution.
- Asking a question, perhaps to clarify a point.

Group communication in formal meetings is usually written down as minutes of the proceedings. Checking that the minutes are accurate, which usually takes place at the next meeting, is important. You also need to check whether the proceedings are confidential, and how widely the minutes will circulate, and to whom.

Contributions of service users

Arnstein's ladder of citizen participation (1969) is an early theoretical perspective that advocated more service user participation. The ladder portrays the different levels of participation.

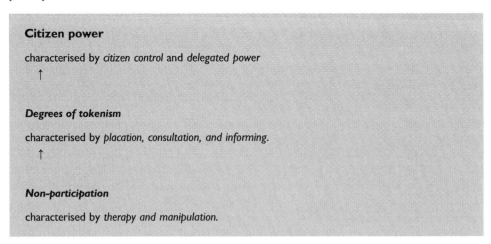

Citizen power

characterised by *citizen control* and *delegated power*

↑

Degrees of tokenism

characterised by *placation, consultation, and informing.*

↑

Non-participation

characterised by *therapy and manipulation.*

Since that early beginning, the development of groups of Experts by Experience (Beresford, 2009, initially mentioned in Chapter 2) has helped make the concept of *personalisation* a powerful driver for change and a strong influence on the ways health practitioners and social workers communicate, both to each other and with service users. *Personalisation* is a concept (discussed also in Chapter 9) that supports choice, independence and people's rights to choose the services they want, by recognising individuals' strengths and preferences. *Personalisation* tries to put individuals at the centre of their own care and support strategies.

Strategies like self-directed support and personal budgets help people to identify their own needs and make choices about how and when they are supported to live their lives. Scourfield (2007) argued that direct payments and individual budgets enable service users to become 'modern citizens' who are clients, consumers, service users, managers, and entrepreneurs. As part of this changed approach, Carr (2011) argues that individuals must have good access to information, advocacy and advice to enable them to make informed decisions. As well, Carr states that there should be an integrated, community-based approach that involves increasing community capacity and using local strategic commissioning. New ways of working will emphasise collaboration (known also as 'co-production') between professional practitioners, managers, and users of services so users will help to design, deliver, and evaluate services.

Personalisation strategy also recognises the contributions of carers and supports their roles, but seeks to help them to live a life beyond their caring roles.

The earlier concept of the *social model* of intervention (Campbell and Oliver, 1996, mentioned in Chapter 3) advocated a power shift between the professional practitioner and the service user towards more service user involvement and decision-making. This change began to soften the impact of professional power on communication and interviewing. Communication between the practitioner and the service user must take note of these new kinds of partnerships between professional practitioners and people who use services, and practise in a facilitative, information-sharing, and consultative manner rather than communicate as a figure of authority.

How service user groups influence professional communication

As discussed in Chapter 3, professional roles have become more challenging as authoritarian attitudes diminish in contemporary society. Media revelations of dishonesty, sexual abuse, and lack of concern for public safety have led to increased public distrust of authority. Because professional practitioners are usually seen as authority figures, they too are less likely to be trusted. Groups known as *Experts by Experience* or *Persons with Lived Experience* are individuals who use health and social care/social work services, or are carers of those persons. They can include, but are not limited to, persons with learning disabilities, autism, mental health conditions, physical impairments, older people, persons who use maternity services, and children and young people.

Beresford (2016) identified four crucial qualities that people who use services want: a *relationship* based on warmth, empathy, reliability and respect; a *social perspective* that sees people's lives in the round, not just the problems; offering *practical as well as emotional support*, and *listening* without judging. These qualities define the characteristics of effective communication. Groups of *Experts by Experience* assist social services, health, housing, and voluntary organisations in planning, reviewing and evaluating service delivery, assist universities in training professional practitioners, and participate as members of boards of trustees. Their contributions are sometimes public, and sometimes anonymous. Social work and the health professions now have active patient and user groups – *Experts by Experience* – who contribute as board and committee members. Their communications are valued parts of service planning and management.

However, counselling and psychotherapy, perhaps because of the individual nature of their practice, apparently do not make widespread use of groups of *Experts by Experience*. Counselling is less engaged, apparently, in the movement to involve clients as equal partners. When preparing this chapter, I contacted a national counselling organisation to ask about client involvement. I was informed that the organisation is not aware of any specific representative client groups, but the mental health organisation Mind does have service user involvement, and NSUN (the National Survivor User Network), which is a network of people living with mental distress, campaigns for change. A welcome development in 2018 was a British Association of Counselling and Psychotherapy journal featuring articles written by clients about their experiences of counselling.

Giving and receiving information: an important kind of communication

Members of the public are now more likely to demand full and accurate information on events that have affected their lives.

Practice example 4.6: *A woman who had experienced a violent marriage and subsequently divorced her husband was devoted to her daughter's two young children. She was devastated when her grandchildren were taken into care because of her daughter's mental health. The children were subsequently placed for adoption, despite her own wish to provide a home for them. She expressed anger because she believed that social services had failed to inform her when the children were placed with an adoptive family. She believed that she had a right to be informed because she was their grandmother who wanted to offer them a home. Because of this failure to acknowledge her love and concern, and to inform her, she said she had lost trust in social services.*

Sometimes professional practitioners inadvertently fail to provide sufficient information to a person requesting services.

Practice example 4.7 *An occupational therapist visited the home of an 85-year-old woman to advise her relatives on the woman's return home from hospital. The woman lived alone, and could no longer walk. The bathroom was upstairs and there was no stair lift. It was not possible to install a stair lift or create a downstairs W.C. The therapist explained that carers would call four times a day. The woman could sleep downstairs in the front room. The therapist said that the woman could use a commode when carers were present and would be fitted with incontinence pads at night. The woman's adult granddaughter, who was present, then asked, 'What will happen if my grandmother has to use the toilet during the day when the carers are not with her?' The therapist had not thought of this.*

The granddaughter had enough confidence to ask a crucial question, but if she had deferred to the power of the professional, the care arrangements would not have been able to maintain the dignity of the patient. This account parallels Vicary and Spencer-Lane's article (2018) about budget impacts on care planning decisions. Their article highlights the example of McDonald v. United Kingdom, a 91-yearold disabled woman who, although not incontinent, was forced to accept incontinence pads because budget reductions meant that insufficient care practitioners were available to meet her personal needs. Although the court determined that the council had violated her right to respect for private and family life, it also acknowledged that the state has discretionary decision-making powers for allocating scarce resources.

Recognising the power of erroneous beliefs that contribute to feelings of guilt and self-blame

Some persons may reveal mistaken beliefs about the causes or consequences of tragic events in their lives. Their feelings are not logical but are deeply felt. These feelings may survive because of fear of criticisms, inhibitions, and the longstanding lack of anyone who listened to them. These persons are likely to have lived in environments where those in authority failed to provide sufficient explanations for what had happened.

> Practice example 4.8 *A middle-aged woman who had lived in poverty confided the reason for her rejection of her daughter many years before. The daughter, at the age of four, was sleeping in the same bed as her six-month-old brother. In the morning, the woman discovered that the baby boy was dead. She never spoke about this, but blamed the daughter, believing that the little girl had rolled on top of the baby and smothered him. She was never informed about the diagnosis of a cot death, so she spent years with a false belief that damaged her ongoing relationship with her remaining child.*
>
> *Questions:* What kind of communication might have prevented this mistaken belief from exerting so much influence in the woman's life and the life of her daughter? How would you respond in the present day to the woman's admission of her feelings?

Practitioners who 'listen with the third ear' (Safran, 2011; Reik, 1983, 1948) can more easily pick up and respond to inner fears and erroneous beliefs. A long-held belief is not surrendered easily, so a gentle approach is needed. Providing full and accurate information can help a person avoid inaccurate beliefs and prevent them from becoming overwhelmed by guilt and self-blame. The woman who blamed her daughter also held deep feelings of guilt.

Implicit and explicit uses of power

Implicit and explicit uses of power (mentioned in Chapter 3) are factors in communication. Professional status invests a practitioner with power to influence how a communication takes place and how the recipient of the communication understands its meaning. Teachers, lawyers, doctors, nurses, social workers, and counsellors convey powerful personae based on their professional roles and their perceptions of the persons who seek help. Professional power is explicit when a judge delivers a verdict in a courtroom, when a doctor makes a diagnosis, or when a social worker removes a child from a parent's care. Implicit power is not always verbalised or evident in a straightforward manner, but persons who observe practitioners' behaviour comprehend this power.

> Practice Example 4.9: *One morning I parked my car on a street of council houses prior to visiting a friend, when I noticed two women in their thirties, dressed in formal business-like clothes, park their*

car ahead of me, get out and proceed briskly and purposefully along the street. One woman carried a brief case, the other carried office files. Both wore lanyards with identification badges around their necks. They spoke to each other in fairly loud tones as they proceeded down the street. I looked at them and surmised that they were on official business. I guessed that they were social workers who were about to visit a family with young children, perhaps to conduct a safeguarding enquiry. I observed their confident, seemingly official demeanour. I did not speak to them and they did not speak to me, but I became aware of their implicit power.

Another example describes how a counsellor failed to gain the trust of a client.

Practice example 4.10 A young woman was being investigated by social services for possible abuse of her young child. She came to an independent charity for counselling. During the counselling, she was often withdrawn, but if asked, said she was fine. The counsellor doubted whether a trusting relationship had been established. After six sessions, the client phoned the charity to say that she wanted to finish counselling. The counsellor reflected that social services had probably instructed the young woman to undertake counselling, and she had felt compelled to come. Counselling, to the young woman, may have seemed part of an oppressive power structure, but she was unable to articulate how she felt.

The counsellor initially was unaware that the young woman feared becoming subject to the counsellor's power, just as she feared social services' power to remove her child. When a practitioner realises that a person who receives services feels compelled to attend and cannot develop trust because of fear of implicit or explicit power, the practitioner is advised to try to bring these feelings into the open in a sensitive accepting manner.

The **heart/soul/emotion** *aspect of practice and the* **head/mind/reason** *aspect of practice*

So far, I have been using a *head/mind/reason* approach in the preceding discussion and providing logical definitions of verbal and non-verbal communication. The next part of the chapter takes a different approach and explores concepts that derive from the *heart/soul/ emotion* aspect of practice, rather than the *head/mind/reason* approach. Practitioners must remember that both approaches are needed. Practitioners communicate constructively when they engage with their own and the person's *heart/soul/emotions*. Three concepts – the *use of relationships* (Biestek, 1992, 1957; Perlman, 1983,1979), *use of self* (Dewane, 2006) and the *art of practice* (England, 1986) were widely used in social work up to the 1970s to help explain the essence of communication between a practitioner and a person. In contemporary practice, Trevithick (2017) is an advocate for relationship-based practice continuing to play an essential part in professional practice.

Changing use of relationships

In the 1950s and 1960s *relationships* (Biestek, 1992, 1957; Hollis, 1972, 1964; Perlman, 1983, 1979 – all based in the USA) were seen as essential tools for developing effective practice. Relationships were used as vehicles for analysing and interpreting persons' behaviour according to Freudian analytic theories (Freud, 1986 edition). Practitioners who used this approach developed roles as implicitly (and sometimes explicitly) powerful professionals. Heavily influenced by psychoanalytic theory, social workers interpreted clients' behaviours as their first priority and overlooked requests for practical help. The classic text, *The Client Speaks* (Mayer and Timms, 1970), exposed the narrowness of this kind of practice, and in effect, helped to end the dominance of the psychoanalytic approach. In Practice example 4.11, the use of a psychoanalytic approach with a group of students sat uneasily with the students' wish to communicate at a more practical level.

> Practice example: 4.11 A group of fifteen social work students on a postgraduate master's degree were required to meet with a psychoanalyst every Monday afternoon at 5 p.m. after a busy day of lectures. Their tutor had explained the purpose of these meetings as adding to their knowledge. The students' attendance was required. Each week the psychoanalyst entered the room, sat down, and was silent. After some minutes, the students became restive. They felt bewildered and annoyed that they were not being offered any knowledge, only silence. The lateness of the afternoon added to their feelings of fatigue and irritation. Eventually, a student asked the psychoanalyst why he was silent. He responded with his interpretation of their anger – the students were said to be angry with him because he represented an authority figure, like a parent, and that this was the relationship they projected onto him. Their emotions were then compared to their own clients' feelings. Although some learning took place, the students remembered their irritation at the silences and the lateness of the day. Ultimately they did not value the sessions because they were not given any opportunity to share their feelings and experiences.

Perhaps the students should have been more tolerant of this approach to learning, but during the time that this encounter took place, other ideas about practice were beginning to take hold. A gradual widening of the concept *of relationship* eroded the acceptance of the professional practitioner's power and use of the analytic approach and moved practice towards more collaborative relationships with people who use services. Over sixty years ago, Hamilton (1951, p. 27), an American social work academic, suggested that a professional relationship should share responsibilities, recognise the person's rights, and accept individual differences. A psychodynamic approach with its implicit professional power continues to be a part of social work practice, but is no longer as dominant an approach as it once was. Contemporary practitioners who practise a psychodynamic approach are likely to explain the *use of relationships* (Biestek, 1992, 1957) as essential for building trust and empowering the person. Rogers' *person-centred* approach (1961, discussed in Chapter 2), emphasises a warm, supportive relationship, and is widely practised across the professions, particularly in counselling and psychotherapy. The person-centred approach integrates well with other practice methods, and can be used alongside psychodynamic and cognitive-behavioural approaches in integrative practice.

Some evidence of changed attitudes towards persons who use services can be found in the Social Work Benchmark Statement (QAA 2016) that states the curriculum requirements for UK social work degrees. Rather than favouring one theoretical approach, the Statement includes a wide range of approaches which unfortunately sometimes obfuscate meaning. The reader who studies the Statement carefully will observe how it recognises that Rogers' person-centred approach has diminished the power of the professional practitioner, and favours sharing decisions with persons who use services and delivering services that promote independence.

Practice example 4.12 from the Social Work Benchmark Statement (QAA, 2016):

1   5. Knowledge, understanding and skills
2   5.1 During their qualifying degree studies in Social Work, students acquire, critically evaluate, apply and integrate knowledge and understanding in......
3   5.6 The leadership, organisation and delivery of Social Work services, which include:
4   xii the development of person-centred services, personalised care, individual budgets and direct payments all focusing upon the human and legal rights of the service user for control, power and self determination.

Social workers (and other professional practitioners) now are expected to use their professional expertise to empower service users, rather than to exercise explicit or implicit power, and their communication skills are meant to convey openness and provide essential information, but sometimes their involvement in socio-legal processes (as discussed in Chapter 3) means that the user of services may feel wary of communicating with a social worker, or with other professional practitioners.

Use of self

Dewane (2006) defines *use of self* operationally as drawing on:

- personality
- belief system(s)
- relational dynamics
- anxiety
- self-disclosure

Use of self can help practitioners develop purposeful communication, if it is used as a tool for increasing self-awareness (Seden, 2005, 1999). Since this concept was developed, professional awareness of injustices and inequalities in persons' lives has increased. Trevithick (2017) broadens the conceptual framework of *self* to include a gendered perspective. *Use of self* suggests that practitioners should develop their own individualised personal style for communicating with others. This does not mean talking volubly about events in one's personal life to a person who seeks help. *Use of self* is a more subtle concept than that, requiring practitioners to practise with self-scrutiny, self-examination, and personal integrity.

Use of self can be both facilitative and a brake on communication. You may find that you sometimes question yourself on how you handled a particular communication – *did I do that right? Did I make a mess of that?* *Use of self* in communication can help persons recognise and understand their own experiences (Howe, 2014). But will success in helping them recognise and understand their experiences always bring about hoped-for changes in a person's life? Not always; practical help may be needed as well.

The art of practice

I have mentioned the 'art' of practice several times in this book.

> *Questions:* What is the 'art of practice'?
>   Does it exist?
>   Can it be taught, or is 'art' an innate, spontaneous quality that has nothing to do with practising a profession?

Freudian-influenced practitioners from previous generations thought of their practice as an 'art'. Hugh England's classic book *Social Work as Art: Making Sense for Good Practice* (1986) is clearly on the side of practice as 'art'. Over time, the growing popularity of evidence-based practice (the 'science' of practice) diminished the credibility of practice as 'art'. When considering Rogers' person-centred approach (discussed in Chapter 2), you may recognise that this theory has to be practised primarily as an *art*. A range of professions adopt *empathy, rapport* and *relationship* as part of communication skills, therefore promoting practice as 'art'. Hood (2018, p. 188) accepts Howe's suggestion (2014, p. 125) that the opposing views of social work as 'art' or 'science' can be resolved by incorporating attributes of both views into a concept of social work as a 'craft'. Hood comments that this notion of social work as 'craft' is achievable only if the 'right' employing organisation employs the 'right' professional practitioners.

Practitioners invest aspects of their personality, individuality, and values in their communication with a person who uses services. A practitioner will learn the different stages of communication (discussed in Chapter 2). The practitioner may plan an interview rationally, using the *head/mind/reason* approach to communication, but is also likely to draw on aspects of their own personality, choosing and combining appropriate techniques in an artful way. Effective communication is achieved by developing your own *art* of practice as well as a logical plan of action.

Importance of reflecting on practice

Practitioners will gain confidence and understanding by reflecting regularly on their practice and identifying what seemed to have gone wrong, what went well, and which events seemed puzzling. The process of doing this can be informal – taking a moment or two each day to jot down a few words or phrases about practice, your questions and issues, and then reviewing these later. Doing this regularly increases practitioners' ability to practise with self-scrutiny, self-examination, and personal integrity. Peer discussion with colleagues can be helpful if the purpose and process is agreed by all. Professional supervision of practice helps prevent possible misuses of power. Supervision at its best should be more than line management – reviewing the necessary nuts and bolts of performing a paid role; it should be used as professional supervision to build perspective, increase self-awareness, and review and develop different communication strategies. Practitioners can communicate more constructively by engaging with their own and the person's emotions, but also by balancing this engagement with self-reflection and professional supervision.

Summary

Communication is an essential tool of practice, and practitioners communicate more effectively when they:

- recognise the importance of all forms of communication (formal and informal, verbal and non-verbal)
- develop their own personal style of communication congruent with their professional role
- build their repertoire of communication skills
- communicate with the *heart/soul/emotion* aspect as well as the *head/mind/reason* aspect of practice
- reflect regularly on their communication
- use professional supervision to ensure their communication is ethical, appropriate, and effective
- evaluate their successes and failures of communication
- are flexible in approach
- value the role of information giving
- recognise how implicit and explicit power affect the person who asks for help
- listen to the voices of *Experts by Experience*
- check whether the person understands your communication

References

Arnstein, S. R. (1969) 'A ladder of citizen participation in the USA', *Journal of the American Institute of Planners*, Volume 35: 216–224.

Beresford, P. (2009) *Compass think piece 47: whose personalisation?*Compass: London.

Beresford, P. (2016) *All our welfare: towards participatory social policy.* Policy Press: Bristol.

Biestek, F. (1992, 1957) *The Casework Relationship.* Routledge: London.

Campbell, J. and Oliver, M. (1996) *Disability politics: understanding our past, changing our future.* Routledge: London.

Carr, Sarah (2011) *Personalisation A Rough Guide. Adult Services SCIE Guide 47.* Social Care Institute for Excellence: London.

Dewane, Claudia J. (2006) 'Use of self: a primer revisited', *Clinical Social Work Journal*, Volume 34, Issue 4, Winter, pp. 543–558.

England, Hugh (1986) *Social Work As Art: Making Sense for Good Practice.* Allen & Unwin: London.

Freud, S. (1986 edition) *The Essentials of Psycho-Analysis* (selected by Anna Freud) Penguin: London.

Hamilton, G. (1951) *Theory and Practice of Social Casework.* 2nd Edition. Columbia University Press: New York.

Hollis, F. (1972 edition) *Casework: A Psychosocial therapy.* 2nd Edition, revised, Random House, New York.

Hollis, Florence. (1964) *Casework. A Psychosocial Therapy.* McGraw Hill: New York.

Hood, Rick (2018) *Complexity in Social Work.* Sage: London.

Howe, D. (2014) *The Compleat Social Worker.* Basingstoke: Palgrave Macmillan.

Jonassen, David, Davidson, Mark, Collins, Mauri, Campbell, John, and Bannan Haag, Brenda (2009, 1995) 'Constructivism and Computer-Mediated Communication in Distance Education', *American Journal of Distance Education*, Volume 9, Issue 2, pp. 7–26. published online 24 September 2009.

Mayer, J. and Timms, N. (1970) *The Client Speaks.* Routledge & Kegan Paul: London.

Perlman, H. H. (1983, 1979) *Relationship: The Heart of Helping People*. University of Chicago Press: Chicago.

*Plain English Campaign (2018)*http://www.plainenglish.co.uk. Accessed 10 June 2018.

QAA Quality Assurance Agency (2016) *Social Work Benchmark Statement*. QAA: Gloucester.

Reik, Theodor (1948, 1983) *Listening with the Third Ear: The Inner Experience of a Psychoanalyst*. Farrar Strauss and Giroux: New York.

Rogers, C. R. (1961) *On Becoming a Person*. Constable: London.

Safran, Jeremy D. (2011) 'Theodor Reik's Listening with the Third Ear and the Role of Self-Analysis in Contemporary Psychoanalytic Thinking'. *The Psychoanalytic Review*, Volume 98. Foreshadowing the Present: the Legacies of Theodor Reik, pp. 2015–2216.

Scourfield, P. (2007) 'Social care and the modern citizen: client, consumer, service user, manager and entrepreneur', *The British Journal of Social Work*, Volume 37, Issue 1: pp 17–22.

Seden, Janet(2005, 1999) *Counselling Skills in Social Work Practice*. 2ndEdition. Open University Press:London.

Trevithick, P. (2017) The 'Self' and the 'Use of Self' in Social Work: A Contribution to the Development of a Coherent Theoretical Framework, *The British Journal of Social Work*. Oxford University Press, 28 November 2017.

Vicary, S. and Spencer-Lane, T. (2018) 'Why budget limits can impact on care planning decisions', *Professional Social Work*, British Association of Social Workers: Birmingham. September 2018, p. 36.

Chapter 5

Interviewing skills

What is an *interview*?

An interview is a formal type of communication where people meet face-to-face (but sometimes through webcam internet contact) for discussion and questioning to achieve specified outcomes.

Aims and outcomes of interviews

Depending on the specific organisational context, interviews are designed to attain specific aims and outcomes. I have chosen to focus on situations that are shared across the social work, counselling, and health professions. Interviews conducted within these professions aim to achieve some of the following outcomes:

- establish the facts of a situation
- evaluate a situation
- exchange ideas and views
- gather evidence to help make future decisions
- address and resolve issues

In an educational setting, the interview's purpose might be to:

- select students for a professional course
- orally examine a student regarding a topic of professional knowledge
- establish whether plagiarism or misconduct has taken place

Employers use interviews to:

- select an applicant for employment, promotion or a volunteer role
- determine whether an employee's behaviour is inadequate or breaches ethical standards
- appraise an employee
- terminate employment

Conducting job interviews: the role of interview panels

During an interview, one or more persons will form an interview panel to conduct the interview. A named chairperson will be a member of the panel and will introduce and conclude the interview. The panel members are likely to be senior managers, practitioners, business administrators, and service user/patient/client/carer representatives. (An interview conducted by more than one person can help avert unconscious bias for or against an applicant.) The interviewee answers the questions posed by the panel, and will have an opportunity at the end to pose their own questions. A significant and relatively recent development is the inclusion of service users/patients/clients as participants on panels for job selection or for selection of students for qualifying professional courses.

Communication before and during the interview

Arranging the layout of the interview room and managing the process in a manner that helps rather than hinders communication is an essential requirement. For example:

- ensure that the applicant is informed in writing about the interview process, whether an informal prior gathering and/or a candidate presentation will take place, and the exact timings of the process.
- avoid placing the applicant in a position where the sun will shine in their eyes, and the resulting glare will obscure their vision.
- try to ensure that no extraneous noise is heard within the room, and that the acoustics of the room are good.
- panel members should speak slowly and ensure the interviewee can hear them.
- the applicant's position in front of the interview panel must not be at a lower level than the panel members.
- clearly display the interview panel's names and job roles so that the applicant knows who is asking the questions.
- if this is not possible, the applicant should be given a written list of the interview panel's names and roles.

Format of the recruitment process

A formal interview may be only one part of the recruitment process, which begins with designing the job description and the required competences for the job, advertising the position, agreeing the application form, drawing up the short list of applicants, and planning the interview process.

A formal interview may be preceded by the applicant giving a brief presentation on a pre-agreed topic. When this is a required part of the process, each applicant must be informed in writing beforehand about the topic, the management and timing of the presentation, the persons who will comprise the audience, and the facilities for presentation.

Some interviews are preceded by *informal gatherings* where the applicants are invited to mingle with the staff and the interview panel. Afterwards, the staff's impressions of the applicants are sometimes fed back to the interview panel before the formal interview.

When this occurs, the applicant should always be informed beforehand that this kind of feedback will be sought. It would be unethical to gather feedback when candidates have not been forewarned that this process will be part of the interview.

Selecting and informing the successful applicant

Following the interview, the panel's task is to select the most suitable applicant. The chair may begin by asking panel members whether they think all the applicants are 'appointable' or not. Sometimes this feedback makes use of numerical scoring of different characteristics and skills. This process may eliminate some candidates from further consideration. Then each panel member is given an opportunity to express their preferences for a particular candidate and why, with evidence based on the candidate's job application and performance at interview. This process usually identifies the applicant who will be offered the job. Sometimes the panel may decide that none of the applicants are suitable and decline to make an appointment. Customs vary about how and when applicants are informed. When I chaired university interview panels to appoint social work, social policy and health lecturers, it was customary to phone the applicants that evening, beginning with a job offer to the preferred applicant. The applicant was expected to say yes or no at that point. A designated salary grade was usually mentioned, and if the applicant was not happy with this, they were expected to discuss the matter at this point. The panel chair then would phone the other applicants to tell them they had not been appointed, and would offer to provide constructive feedback. Being informed that you were considered appointable and being given some positive feedback can encourage an applicant's further efforts, and on more than one occasion at subsequent professional gatherings I came into contact with practitioners who had not been appointed on that initial occasion but who told me they valued the feedback they were given, and that had encouraged them to make further attempts which met with success.

   This is one example of how the process could be managed. Other employers may choose not to telephone applicants but write to the preferred applicant with a job offer, thus delaying the process of finalising the appointment.

References

Employers use references to confirm a job appointment. The reference provides a view of the applicant's past experience. Making a job offer is usually provisional until satisfactory references are received. Should the panel be informed of the content of the references before an interview? In general, references are held back until after the interview. Not all references may have been received at the date of the interview.

Equal Opportunities protocols

Equal Opportunities protocols now shape the structure and process of a job interview, but protocols may be interpreted differently. Skills for Care's website, (www.skillsforcare. org.uk/valuesandbehaviours, accessed 18 June 2018) contains a summary of information on Equal Opportunities and interviewing. Interviewers should complete Equal Opportunities training for interview selection processes before conducting an interview.

The Equality Act 2010 states that employers should not treat one job applicant worse than another because of age, disability, gender, reassignment of gender, marriage and civil partnership, pregnancy, maternity, race, religion, belief, sex, and sexual orientation, all of which are *protected characteristics*. The Act also states that employers should not treat a job applicant *worse*

- because they are associated with a person who has a protected characteristic
- because you incorrectly think they have a protected characteristic

or treat a job applicant

- *unfavourably* because of something connected to their disability where you cannot show that what you are doing is objectively justified
- *bully* or *victimise* them because they have complained about discrimination or helped someone else complain

or

- do something which has a *worse* impact on a job applicant and on other people who share a particular characteristic than on people who do not have that characteristic

or

- *harass* a job applicant

Best practice for interviewing

Skills for Care highlights what it considers best practice for interviewing, based on the advice of the Equality and Human Rights Commission (www.equalityhumanrights.com) so that an employer can demonstrate that their interviewing process is consonant with legal requirements. This requires employers to

- ask applicants beforehand whether they need adjustments to the interview process to allow them to attend and participate fully
- make *reasonable adjustments* to the process for these applicants
- be flexible with dates and times
- focus on the skills, qualities and experience required for the job
- ask questions based on the job description and the competences set out for the job

Employers should NOT

- ask questions about a protected characteristic, unless these relate to the job
- ask about health, disability or sickness records
- make instant, personal or unfair judgements about an applicant because of their protected characteristics

Questions for the applicant

Before current Equal Opportunities legislation was introduced, the public's collective consciousness of inequality was minimal. Job interviews frequently asked women whether they were married, pregnant, whether they had children and how many. Both men and women were asked their age and their country of origin. These kinds of questions were shaped by stereotypical assumptions, for example, concerns that:

- *an older applicant might be unable to learn new tasks, and would feel uncomfortable working with younger people.*
- *a woman might become pregnant, or have family responsibilities that make her unable to manage the job responsibilities.*
- *An individual from another country would not be able to cope with the requirements of the job.*

Questions about age, disability, identity, and assumptions about gender roles are now considered discriminatory and must not be asked.

Set questions and supplementary questions

Interview panels often use pre-determined *set* questions. Each panel interviewer will be assigned a particular question to ask, and will use exactly the same words when posing their question to each applicant. Panels may believe that this procedure ensures that the interview accords with Equal Opportunities, but the applicant may perceive the panel's manner as conveying little enthusiasm or animation. Panels should consider how they might avoid the extremes of a rigid questioning process. The Equality and Human Rights Commission (2018) argues that it is a myth that interviewers must ask the same questions of each applicant. Similarly, although some interview panels may argue that *supplementary questions* are not permissible under Equal Opportunities legislation, the Commission says it is possible to ask follow-up questions that relate to something the applicant has just said, but you should focus on the same subject areas for each applicant to avoid unlawful discrimination.

Preparing for a job interview where you are the applicant

Sometimes instead of interviewing others, you are the job applicant and need to prepare for an interview. This may be an *external* interview (when you are not employed by the organisation) or an *internal* interview (where you are already an employee but want to change your role). An internal interview should be as meticulous and adherent to Equal Opportunities protocols as an external interview.

When you are the applicant, study the job description and the required competences, and think about how your previous employment and education might equip you to demonstrate these. Perhaps you may not feel confident, but try to act 'as if' you are, whilst avoiding making extravagant claims about your skills. It may help if you prepare a specially constructed *curriculum vitae* mapped against the job requirements for your own use in preparation. You might want to rehearse how you will respond to the probable questions. You can usually predict what some of the questions will be:

- *Why do you want this job?*
- *What skills and knowledge do you bring?*
- *How will you tackle the requirements of the job?*
- *Please give an example of how you would....*

As well as ensuring that you possess the requisite competences for the job, the panel will want to discover whether as an employee, you would be a cooperative team member who is enthusiastic and committed to the job. Despite nervousness, try to stay calm, and thank the panel for their time at the end of the interview.

Avoiding disillusionment

Sometimes an interview reveals inadvertent information about the workings of an organisation that may cause you to doubt whether you would be happy working there. Trust these feelings! The purpose of job interviews is not just to test your abilities, but to provide you with an opportunity to learn more about the organisation and decide whether you really want to work there.

> Interview Examples:
> A panel member persistently confuses the name of the applicant's university (which was clearly stated on the application form) with the name of a commercial firm.
> A panel member interrupts an applicant who is answering a question about safeguarding and tells the applicant that the answer is wrong. Then the panel chair intervenes and tells the panel member that the applicant's response is correct.

These examples are unlikely to build the applicant's confidence in the organisation.

Preparing for informal gatherings and presentations before a formal interview

As an applicant, you are advised to be aware that every aspect of a selection process requires careful preparation and concentration. As soon as you enter the building where the interview will take place, approach a reception desk, and walk down a corridor towards the interview room, you need to maintain your focus on your goal. Some applicants confide their nervousness or reveal feelings of irritation or impatience to a person at the reception desk. Applicants may become inadvertently indiscreet during an informal gathering that precedes the formal interview. Try to be your 'professional self' throughout the entire process.

When you make a presentation, you need to appear confident and knowledgeable, and you can achieve this if you prepare ahead of time.

- *Don't rush or gabble – speak slowly and ensure you can be heard.*
- *Effectively use appropriate equipment to display your presentation.*
- *Avoid cluttering a presentation screen with too many symbols, cartoons, and pictorial representations.*
- *Do not read constantly from notes that you hold in your hand. If you have to refer to notes, have them on a table and only glance at them from time to time.*
- *Include only a few lines of information on each screen.*
- *Provide additional details in your vocal commentary.*
- *Prepare and distribute a handout that contains more detail.*
- *Ensure that your use of the English language is accurate.*
- *Proof read any written or displayed material carefully and correct any spelling or grammatical errors.*

Online interviews

Increasingly, interviews may be conducted online via Skype. Although undoubtedly convenient, less time consuming and more cost-effective to organise, the internet process can make communication between the participants seem stilted and overly formal. It is best to rehearse beforehand how you, as an applicant, will present yourself. The interview panel also need to make an effort to communicate clearly.

Interviewing a service user/patient/client

Examples of conducting a professional interview include (but are not limited to) making an assessment, a diagnosis, and gathering evidence for a formal purpose (Kadushin and Kadushin, 1997).

- Be clear about your purpose and role when you conduct a professional interview.
- Ensure that you are familiar with your organisation's policy on confidentiality
- In every aspect of an interview, apply principles of good practice as you listen to and speak with a person who presents a particular situation that may be troubling them.
- Show *rapport* and *empathy* (discussed in Chapter 3).
- Try to set the interviewee at ease.
- Be aware of attitudes of *intersectionality* unwittingly sabotaging the process.

Steps of an interview

The first step of every interview is to clarify the reasons for meeting together.

The second step is to clarify the extent and limits of confidentiality, and why and when confidentiality may have to be breached – e. g. when a safeguarding issue arises. You will also need to explain how the information you gather will be recorded and used. In addition to direct questions, facilitative comments can encourage discussion such as, 'could you please give me an example'; or 'do you feel that...'

Bringing along a supporter or spokesperson

When person who is being interviewed is a client or an employee who is facing a disciplinary hearing, they may wish to bring along a supporter. A supporter may not participate directly, but will act as a witness and an encouraging presence. On other occasions, an individual with a physical impairment may ask to have a spokesperson who can assist in articulating the individual's views. The individual should seek permission ahead of time if they would like to bring along a supporter or spokesperson.

Developing a professional interviewing style

Your manner when you are conducting an interview should reflect your professional integrity and regard for those you are interviewing. Don't gaze at a computer screen, look at the participant(s) frequently but do not appear to stare at them. Remember that individuals from some cultures may be reluctant to look at you directly. If you are a social worker or a counsellor, and the interview's purpose is to assess the person's situation and need for help, you probably will be required to complete a pro-forma that asks detailed information about the person. Explain why you are asking for this information and the purposes for which it will be used. If you are a health practitioner who has to make a diagnosis or treat the patient, ask for information in a succinct planned sequence.

The stages of a professional interview resemble those of good communication, as discussed in Chapter 2. You will want to check whether the person understands what has been said. (Understanding is more easily achieved if you avoid jargon and acronyms.) It is wise not to change the subject quickly, because that can be distracting to the person.

Silences may occur, and you may feel you are getting nowhere, but ask yourself what the silences mean. The person may find revealing themselves emotionally difficult or you may have touched on a topic they find very upsetting to discuss. You may be interviewing a person who really does not want to participate – try to find out why. The person's distress may evoke an inner disturbed reaction in yourself – but try to maintain your professional demeanour, accept the person as they are, but do not offer too much reassurance at an early stage. When you reach the end of the interview, summarise the discussion, check again for understanding, and discuss possible choices for the future.

Group interviews

Some situations may require group interviews. An example of a setting where this might occur is in the quality assurance processes of university education. Approval processes for new professional courses usually require professional approval by the profession's regulatory body, with a panel sent to the campus to conduct group interviews. Panel members will normally meet with a group of experts by experience and carers and ask their views about the course and the university. The same requirements for good communication are necessary here – explain the meeting's purpose, introduce yourself clearly, avoid jargon and acronyms, speak slowly, and check for mutual understanding.

One or more panel members may ask the questions, and another member is delegated to note the responses.

Summary

The characteristics and purposes of interviews span the professions, and the required skills are similar, although the purposes and desired outcomes may differ for each profession. This similarity encourages the development of multi-professional practice. Greater objectivity may be achieved if an interviewing panel includes a user of services and a practitioner from a different profession. Interviewing takes place within professional power structures, but contemporary trends in health and social work practice suggest an increase in using more facilitative attempts to engage with and empower the person, so that their participation is more assured. Equal Opportunities legislation and patient/service user/client/carer groups continue to modify authoritarian power structures and enable the patient/client/service user to have more 'voice' to express their concerns.

References

Equality and Human Rights Commission (2018) *Advice and Guidance* www.equalityhumanrights. com. Website accessed 7 September 2018.

Kadushin, Alfred and Kadushin, Goldie (1997) *The Social Work Interview: A Guide for Human Services Professionals*. Columbia University Press: New York.

Skills for Care (2018) 'Recruitment and retention. Values and behaviours-based recruitment, Equal Opportunities and interviewing' www.skillsforcare.org.uk/Documents/Recruitment-and-reten tion/Values-and-behaviours-based-recruitmenEqual-opportunities-and-interviewing.pdf. Website accessed 8 August 2018.

Conceptual themes for communicating and interviewing in different practice situations

Communication skills for specific professional roles

On a day-to-day basis, you will use your communication skills in situations related to your professional role. A broad overview might assert that social workers communicate with individuals who experience social problems and deprivation; counsellors communicate with individuals who experience emotional and mental problems; and health care professionals communicate with individuals who experience physical and mental health issues. In general terms, there is truth in this assertion, because each profession claims particular knowledge and skills as its own. Communication skills, however, span the professions and are the basic tools of every practitioner. Although the focus and desired outcomes of interventions differ from profession to profession, these professions draw on similar communication skills.

Factors that influence individual well-being

How can a practitioner begin to communicate more effectively? First, you might consider how a mix of psychological, physical and social factors influences individual well-being.

- psychological factors include emotional states: anxiety, fear, sadness, and depression, but also joy and contentment
- physical factors include illnesses like cancer, heart disease, and diabetes, but also physical activities of participation in healthy living activities
- social factors include homelessness, poverty, a history of abuse, violence, and loneliness, but also a sense of achievement and belonging

(You will be able to think of many additional examples.)

These three categories of psychological, emotional, and social factors could be considered separately, but separating them would deny their conjoined existence in each individual. Specialist professional roles try to help individuals deal with issues that arise from these three factors. Different professions tend to focus on different factors in this mix, but professional practitioners need to start by considering the essence of the whole human being – their humanity – not a segmented example of social problems, ill health, or mental illness.

To use communication skills effectively, practitioners from different professions should recognise aspects of people's problems that require a commonality of expertise.

Practitioners engage with individuals whose health problems may trigger psychological problems, whose social problems may exacerbate their mental health problems, and whose mental health problems may affect their physical health. How can a professional practitioner recognise and respond to the *whole* of a person, not just to the aspect that falls within their own expertise?

> **Practice Example 6.1** *A male patient visited his GP complaining of persistent headaches. The GP questioned him about their frequency and intensity, and was about to prescribe some medication and refer the patient for tests, when the patient suddenly confided that he was in debt, he had not paid his rent for several months, and next week he and his family would be evicted. Suddenly the situation looked very different. The GP realised that the patient's most immediate problem lay outside his professional remit.*
>
> *Question:* **What should the doctor do?**

If the GP practice employs a social worker, a referral could be made to the social worker who can liaise with the housing authority and negotiate repayment of the arrears to stave off the eviction. But currently it is more likely that the appropriate expertise to resolve this issue will lie outside the medical practice. The dilemma for specialist professions is that, whilst society needs their specialist expertise, their separately organised specialisms tend to overlook the 'whole' of a person, requiring a person to wait for a separate referral to an additional specialism.

How social, personal, and spiritual contexts influence communication

Social and personal contexts exert strong influences on people's sense of well-being, and the skilled practitioner will recognise these in their communication with patients/clients/service users. The person you are trying to help will benefit from your acknowledgement of the impact of personal and social contexts on their lives. Social contexts may include poverty, homelessness, disability, violence, gender and sexuality issues, and loss. Personal contexts include broken relationships, stigma, prejudice and social isolation, and draw also on the ideas of ecological contexts (Bronfenbrenner, 1979).

Spiritual contexts (Crisp, 2017) also enter into communication. Spirituality is part of the human condition. Deriving from concepts of the 'spirit', spirituality usually refers to a higher consciousness, or to meanings that cannot be proven by logic. Spirituality questions what is real and significant, and searches for understanding. It is often, but not always, linked to religious belief. As a practitioner, you don't have to be a religious believer, or an expert, but you may need to acknowledge the unknowability of some aspects of human life and recognise that many individuals search for meaning in different ways (Frankl, 2014, 2011, 1969). Their spiritual contexts seek to be heard. When a person begins to tell you their spiritual concerns, do not respond with a statement about your own beliefs or lack of beliefs. Some social workers and counsellors feel the need to state their own faith or lack of faith when a person begins to discuss their religious or spiritual beliefs. This is intrusive and turns the focus away from the client towards yourself.

The wise practitioner acknowledges, rather than ignores, these three contexts – social, personal, and spiritual. Be empathetic, non-judgemental, and listen. Be 'with' the person in the Rogerian sense (1961). The practitioner's role is to communicate by offering acceptance of the individual's personhood – *unconditional positive regard* (Rogers, 1961).

Constructive practice

Individual lives and well-being are influenced not only by the psychological factors of emotions, feelings and inner drives and by social and environmental factors, but also by the ways that people search for meaning (Frankl, 2014) through constructing their ideas and opinions about the significance of particular events. Robert Neimeyer, a psychologist, who draws on Kelly's personal constructs theory (1955), has written extensively about constructive theories and therapeutic techniques. According to Neimeyer (2009, p. 1) 'every emerging perspective repackages the wisdom of earlier thinkers [and] adds its own insights and innovations'. Neimeyer draws on approaches from other models but adds his own distinctive touches. He uses person-centred theory to form and sustain a therapeutic relationship, and draws on gestalt theory (Perls, 1969) by using the *Empty Chair* technique, where the grieving individual is invited to speak to an empty chair that represents the lost person. This approach can be effective in situations of loss to enable a personal relationship to become meaningful in a different, reconstructed way.

Neimeyer (2009, p. 59) also uses gestalt theory to emphasise the *presence* of the therapist; he critiques the modern trend for 'rule-governed, reliable and replicable' interventions (Held, 1995) 'bleached of the idiosyncrasy' of individual variation, advocating instead 'the inherent individuality of therapy and its necessary tailoring to the immediacy of the encounter between *this* therapist working with *this* client at this moment of emergent understanding of the problem before them' (p. 59). Although his statement refers to therapy, these principles also apply to communication and interviewing skills. Neimeyer's practice illustrates the drawing together of different theoretical approaches in a manner suitable for addressing contemporary issues.

The ecological approach

Ecological counselling (Cook, 2013; Shallcross, 2013) is a largely American approach to counselling that fits with the belief that social and personal contexts influence people's lives. Ecological theory developed as part of the work of Uri Bronfenbrenner (1979, discussed also in Chapter 2), who drew on the theories of Kurt Lewin (1948). Bronfenbrenner conceptualised different layers of relationships: close, one-to-one relationships (micro-level); family and friends relationships (meso-level), societal and employment relationships (macro-level) and relationships to the wider society (endo-level). Throughout these levels, the individual engages with different value systems, life goals, and spiritual beliefs, and searches for meaning. Professional practitioners who wish to improve their communication skills will benefit from acknowledging the different ecological contexts that shape personal identity.

The search for meaning

Viktor Frankl's logotherapy theorises that the *search for meaning* (2014; 2011, 1969) constitutes a significant motivating force for human behaviour. Consonant with

Bronfenbrenner's ecological framework, the individual who searches for meaning will develop a relationship with the wider society in which they live as well as engaging in dyadic, intimate relationships. Ecological structures influence individual life goals, values, and beliefs, and are an integral part of the search for meaning.

Encouraging personal narratives

A personal narrative is the communicated story that an individual tells as part of their search for meaning. A professional practitioner can enable an individual to tell their story if first they build trust. As trust grows, the individual will share more of their story. The practitioner must listen carefully to the person, and accept their faults and fears. Gradually the practitioner and the individual will jointly recognise the social and personal contexts that shape the individual's life, and discover the meaning the individual gives to significant life events. This narrative will also reveal the extent to which the individuals perceive themselves as being subject to oppressive power. The personal narrative can reveal frightening beliefs and fears.

> *Practice example 6.2: A mother, whose five-year-old daughter experienced several episodes of fits and was diagnosed with epilepsy, appeared to distance herself from her daughter. Speaking in a frightened, hesitant manner, she said 'my daughter's not the same person – she has changed – she is possessed'.*
>
> *Question: What would you say to the mother?*

A helpful response would acknowledge the mother's fears about her daughter's condition, encourage the mother to express her feelings, avoid judging her, provide accurate information about managing the medical condition, and express belief in her caring abilities to try to reduce her fears. You may not have time to speak at length about her underlying beliefs, but some well-chosen words can communicate hope and support. Some therapists practise narrative therapy (White, 2007), engaging in biographical life stories with the client.

'On-the-spot' counselling and crisis intervention

Practice Example 6.2 is an example of *on-the-spot counselling*, a concept developed by Ainsworth and Fulcher (1982) for their Practice Curriculum for Group Care. Although developed many years ago for a specific group of non-professional staff in social care, *on-the-spot counselling* is relevant to contemporary professional practice. This approach is not a full-blown counselling approach, but a type of *crisis intervention* technique (Lindemann, 1944).

A crisis situation occurs when an individual's reactions to events result in a sense of being overwhelmed and unable to cope. The individual may become anxious, confused, incoherent, angry, depressed, may threaten violence or suicide, or exhibit numbness and denial that are part of the stages of loss and bereavement (Kubler-Ross, 1969). In crisis intervention (Roberts, 2004; O'Hagan, 1986, 1991) the practitioner intervenes as swiftly as possible after the crisis reveals itself, and takes control briefly to enable an individual to reduce anxiety, begin to think rationally, and find coping strategies to overcome the crisis.

One of the most important requirements for the practitioner is to be able to identify a crisis reaction and deal with it by first adopting a structured approach and then appropriately timing the handing back of control to the individual. *Crisis intervention* is short term and intensive and tries to ensure the safety of the individual by calling for additional help when required. *On-the-spot counselling* is consonant with some of the characteristics of crisis intervention because its aim is to reduce stress by responding to an individual's unexpected casually expressed concerns that may be voiced at seemingly inappropriate times. Practitioners will encounter crises and will be called on to respond. The practitioner must be able to identify crisis reactions, deal with them by adopting a structured approach which may require calling for additional professional services to help keep the individual safe, and then (when and if it is feasible) use appropriate timing to hand back control to the individual.

The art of *on-the-spot counselling* is demonstrated by the empathetic brief response of a practitioner who recognises that a person wants to share a significant powerful emotion at an inappropriate time, perhaps at the end of a meeting or when saying goodbye. What does the practitioner do then? You don't have the time to begin a long counselling session. Do you send the person away and say '*I don't have time to discuss this today. Please make an appointment*'? Your ability to recognise the person's desperation and respond appropriately needs an immediate, succinct, and purposeful response. You need to acknowledge the person's emotion with empathy, indicate that you have understood what has been said, and give a brief appropriate response.

> Practice example 6.3 *A practitioner met with a group of teenagers in a further education college. At the meeting's end, a sixteen-year-old girl from the group approached the practitioner and said 'My aunt's husband told me he is in love with me and we should run away together. He won't let me tell my mother. What should I do?' The practitioner was aware that she had only a few minutes to respond because the girl had to attend a class. Thinking quickly, she said 'You must tell your mother. She will be your mother for the rest of your life and you don't want to lose her. Ask her to handle the situation.' The next week, the girl reported that she had told her mother, who 'sorted out the situation and everything was all right now'.*

The practitioner's response was more directive than usual, illustrating *on-the-spot counselling* that addressed a personal crisis.

Practice issues that span the professions

Separate professional roles will engage with specific practice issues, but some issues span the professions. You may find yourself having to communicate with an individual about:

- lack of confidence
- loss of self-esteem
- self-blame
- loneliness
- lack of acceptance by others
- fear

- a feeling that life has no meaning
- a wish to escape responsibilities

These are a few of the feelings that may be revealed. Other situations are more specific: homelessness, unemployment, violence, debt, or a specific personal crisis. (Practitioners will be able to add other emotions and situations to this list.) Although your primary role may not enable you to engage with these additional emotions and problems in depth, your communication does need to acknowledge the expressed concerns of the *whole* person. A brief empathetic response is better than no response at all.

Attachment theory and resilience

Attachment theory (Bowlby, 1951, 1969) suggests that to gain understanding of present-day adult relationships, the professional practitioner should consider past relationships, particularly relationships of early childhood. Attachment theory helps practitioners understand how communication and interviewing and therapeutic interventions might be impeded by life events of the past. Bowlby (1951, 1969) emphasised the importance of a close mother–child relationship, arguing that lack of attachment in infancy could lead to future difficulties in forming trusting adult relationships – the adult unconsciously fearing the repetition of disastrous past relationships, and therefore avoiding commitments, and repeating the avoidant behaviour learned in childhood.

Resilience theory, 'a capacity, which allows a person, group or community to prevent, minimise or overcome the damaging effects of adversity' (Grotberg, 1997) provides an explanation of why some children and adults use opportunities and develop well whilst others fail to use opportunities that might help them overcome earlier deprivation. A more nuanced finding emerged from research by Werner et al. (1982, 1989) which was a significant longitudinal study of all children born in 1955 on the island of Kauai in Hawaii. The research concluded that four factors enabled some disadvantaged children to become competent adults: resilient children were sociable, active, alert, responsive, and could ask for help when needed; some families had fewer children born at relatively widely spaced intervals; the children established a close bond with at least one caregiver (not necessarily a parent); and they found sources of emotional support outside the family from teachers, youth leaders, and peers. These findings suggest strategies for understanding and responding to the impact of childhood deprivation on adult lives.

Cognitive approaches to communication

Cognitive behavioural therapy (CBT, Beck, 1975) and REBT (Rational Emotive Behavioural Therapy, Ellis, 1975) typify a turn away from the Freudian approach of delving into past relationships over a prolonged period of time. Cognitive approaches emphasise an individual's ability to think through issues in order to alter their thinking about their problems and moderate their emotions.

- Beck's cognitive behavioural therapy (1975) tries to resolve client issues by changing unhelpful thinking patterns that can affect emotions. CBT seeks to identify, analyse and change counter-productive cognitions and behaviours, and asks the client to work actively on changing their negative thought processes, believing that emotional distress is a result of distorted thoughts in a situation. Homework may consist of recording a diary of events relevant to the client's issues, exercises to develop more rational self-beliefs, paying more attention to situational reality, and confronting destructive notions of perfectionism.

- The REBT therapist–client relationship (Ellis, 1975) aims to be supportive and facilitative, by using an empathetic approach and providing support while challenging irrational thoughts. The therapist aims to change beliefs quickly, rather than slowly, by teaching *rational self-acceptance*, but acknowledging that other beliefs from the client's value system may help individuals achieve happiness.
- Mindfulness (Stahl et al., 2014) is a cognitive technique whose steps include intention to change, adopting an open mind, patience, acknowledgement of one's experience as it is, a non-judgemental attitude towards oneself, non-striving or accepting an experience as it is, self-reliance, letting be (learning to 'ride' the experience as it is), self-compassion, and balance and equanimity.
- Constructivist therapy uses cognitive techniques like 'laddering' concerns within a hierarchical chart (Neimeyer, 2009).

Summary

A practitioner who learns to communicate effectively will realise that in most situations more than listening is required. Situations will arise when you may not have the time for a long session, but you need to do something. You have to be able to respond appropriately, sometimes quickly. You have to decide whether the situation is a crisis, whether there is a risk of harm, and whether to take immediate action and call on additional help. You need to learn how to integrate separate issues without losing focus on the most important issues. This chapter suggests that a basis for effective communication involves

- knowledge of the *social and personal contexts* that influence communication
- recognising an individual's *search for meaning*
- *constructing* and *reconstructing* meaning
- communicating effectively and taking appropriate action in *crisis* situations
- using selected *cognitive approaches* to enable individuals to think differently about themselves

Much more could be said about the range of concepts and approaches to communication outlined in this chapter. The practitioner is encouraged to delve deeper and continue their learning on these topics by reflecting on their own experience, using professional supervision, and embarking on continuous formal and informal learning that will help to fill in gaps in knowledge and expertise.

References

Ainsworth, F. and Fulcher, L. (1982) *A Practice Curriculum for Group Care Paper.* 14.2 CCETSW: London.

Beck, A.T. (1975). *Cognitive therapy and the emotional disorders.* International Universities Press: Madison, CT.

Bowlby, J. (1969) *Attachment and Loss, Vol. 1: Attachment.* Basic Books: New York:

Bowlby, J. (1973) *Attachment and Loss, Vol. 2: Separation: Anxiety and anger.* Basic Books: New York.

Bowlby, J. (1980) *Attachment and Loss, Vol. 3: Loss: Sadness and depression.* Basic Books: New York.

Bowlby, J. (1951). *Maternal care and mental health.* World Health Organisation Monograph: Geneva.

Bronfenbrenner, U. (1979) *The Ecology of Human Development.* Harvard University Press: Cambridge, MA:

Cook, Ellen P., (2013) *Understanding People in Context: The Ecological Perspective in Counselling.* American Counselling Association. Wiley: Hoboken, NJ.

Crisp, Beth (ed.) (2017) *The Routledge Handbook of Religion, Spirituality and Social Work.* Routledge: London.

Ellis, A. (1975) *A New Guide to Rational Living.* Wilshire Book Company: Chatsworth, CA.

Frankl, V. (2014) *The Will to Meaning: Foundations and Applications of Logotherapy.* Meridian: London.

Frankl, V. (2011, 1969) *Man's Search for Ultimate Meaning.* Basic Books: Cambridge, MA.

Freud, A. (2018, 1936) *The Ego and the Mechanisms of Defense.* Routledge: Abingdon.

Grotberg, E. (1997) 'The International Resilience Project: Findings from the Research and the Effectiveness of Interventions' in B. Bain et al. (eds), *Psychology and Education in the 21st Century: Proceedings of the 54th Annual Convention of the International Council of Psychologists.* IC Press: Edmonton. pp 118–128.

Held, B.S. (1995) *Back to Reality.* Norton: New York.

Kelly, G.A. (1955*) The Psychology of Personal Constructs.* Routledge: New York.

Kubler-Ross, E. (1969) *On Death and Dying.* Macmillan: New York.

Lewin, Kurt (1948) *Resolving Social Conflicts* Harper: New York.

Lindemann, E. (1944) 'Symptomatology and management of acute grief', *American Journal of Psychiatry*, Volume 101, pp. 141–148.

Neimeyer, Robert A. (2001) (ed.) *Meaning Reconstruction and the Experience of Loss.* American Psychological Association: Washington, D. C. pp. 1–9.

Neimeyer, Robert A. (2009) *Constructivist Psychotherapy.* Routledge: London.

O'Hagan, K. (1986) *Crisis Intervention in Social Services.* Macmillan: London.

O'Hagan, K. (1991) 'Crisis Intervention in Social Work' in J. Lishman (ed.), *A Handbook of Theory for Practice Teachers in Social Work.* Jessica Kingsley: London.

Parkes, Colin Murray (2013, 1972) *Bereavement: Studies of Grief in Adult Life.* Routledge: London (with Prigerson, Holly G.)4th Edition.

Perls, F. S. (1969) *Gestalt Therapy Verbatim.* Real People Press: Lafayette, CA.

Roberts, A. R. (2004) *Crisis Intervention Handbook: Assessment, Treatment, and Research.* 2nd Edition. Oxford University Press: Oxford.

Rogers, C. (1951) *Client-Centered Therapy: Its Current Practice, Implications and Theory.* Constable: London.

Rogers, C. R. (1961) *On Becoming a Person.* Constable: London.

Shallcross, Lynne (2013) 'Building a More Complete Client Picture', *Counseling Today* American Counseling Association, pp. 30–40.

Silverman, P. R. and Klass, D. (1996) 'Introduction: What's the problem?' in D. Klass, P.R. Silverman and S.L. Nickman (eds), *Continuing Bonds.* Taylor and Francis: Washington, DC pp. 4–27.

Silverman, P. R. and Nickman, S.L. (1996) 'Concluding thoughts' in D. Klass, P.R. Silverman and S.L. Nickman (eds) *Continuing Bonds.* Taylor and Francis: Washington, D. C., pp. 345–355.

Stahl, R., Meleo-Meyer, F., Koerbel, L. (2014) *A Mindfulness-Based Stress Reduction Workbook for Anxiety.* New Harbinger Publications: Oakland, CA.

Stroebe, M. S. and Schut, H. (1999) 'The dual process model of coping with bereavement: Rationale and description'. *Death Studies*, Volume 23, pp. 197–211.

Stroebe, M. S. and Schut, H. (2001) 'Meaning making in the dual process model of coping with bereavement' in R.A. Neimeyer (ed.), *Meaning Reconstruction and the Experience of Loss.* American Psychological Association: Washington, D. C. pp. 55–73.

Werner, Emmy E. (1982, 1989) 'Children of the Garden Island', *Scientific American*. Volume 260, Issue 4 (April), pp. 106–111.

White, Michael (2007) *Maps of Narrative Practice*. W.W. Norton: New York.

Worden, W. (2002) *Grief Counseling and Grief Therapy: A handbook for the mental health practitioner*. 3rd Edition. Springer: New York.

Chapter 7

Information-giving as a means of communication

The definition and purpose of information-giving

Information-giving is not the same as providing advice and 'telling' someone what to do. The purpose of providing a range of information within a helping process can be characterised as attempts to

- expand the range of choices by providing a variety of relevant information, from which individuals can choose their future courses of action
- help individuals draw on wider ranges of knowledge when they make decisions
- build confidence in their ability to decide what to do in given situations

Different professional approaches to information-giving

Professions differ on their views about providing information. The health professions are more used to giving direct advice (physicians and nurses): their patients expect a diagnosis of being told what is wrong, and then being given advice on what to do. More recently, for some health issues, professional practitioners within the health professions will provide an explanation, suggest some possible ways forward, but then ask the patient what choice of treatment they might prefer.

> Practice Example 7.1 An older patient visited his general practitioner six months after the death of his wife, worried about his continued experience of feeling periods of extreme fatigue. The GP asked about his general health and well-being and about the medication he was taking. She suggested that she could give him a stronger anti-depressant, refer him for counselling, and/or arrange for some blood tests to determine whether there was some underlying unknown cause of the fatigue. She asked him which he preferred – 'what would you like me to do?' After some discussion, the man said that he did not want more medication, did not want counselling, but he did want blood tests, because he was worried that he might be developing some undetected health condition.

Social workers traditionally have been taught to practise within a Rogerian person-centred theoretical stance (Rogers, 1961), to offer a 'listening ear', and adopt a therapeutic relationship-based approach, but this style does not sit well alongside their authoritative socio-legal responsibilities for safeguarding. The public's view of social work is perhaps biased by media outcries that portray social workers as snatching children away from their parents and putting older people into residential homes against their will. Social workers have to strike a balance between their supportive therapeutic roles and their more authoritarian roles. A conflict of identity can result from the pull between two extremes.

Counsellors are perhaps most likely to be wary of giving information to a client. The 'listening ear' approach tends to dominate their techniques. They do not see themselves as being authoritarian. They may fear that information-giving may be another name for telling an individual what to do – a big 'no-no' for counsellors. Yet counsellors do recognise that their clients sometimes need information about other services and other sources of help. This may be called 'sign-posting' to other agencies.

How does a professional practitioner 'sign-post'? I would argue that simply mentioning the existence of a national organisation – for example, Alcoholics Anonymous or the Carers Federation – may not be sufficient. The person who receives a service from you may lack confidence about approaching new organisations and may not be used to searching out local offices of national charities. Your 'sign-posting' may need to include some brief information-giving about local services, what kind of services they provide, and how to approach them, with the proviso that this information is not intended to compel a client to use these services, but simply to give them more possible choices to consider.

Multiple problems and shared confidentiality

One of the issues of offering help to an individual is that you may discover multiple problems not only within the client's situation, but within the situations of other family members that affect your client and impede your client's recovery. What do you do when this happens? It is not always feasible to sign-post outward to other agencies and leave it at that; potentially, individual members of one family could be clients of professional practitioners from several organisations each with different purposes. The issue of *shared confidentiality* comes to the fore. When several agencies are involved, the question arises: how should they communicate with each other so they avoid duplicating services and working at cross purposes from one other? Joint meetings at regular intervals can help develop effective shared strategies for exchanging information. This means that certain confidential aspects about a client must be shared within agreed interagency policies for shared confidentiality, and the client must be informed and give permission for certain information to be shared.

Practice Example 7.2 *Sometimes one agency may offer several programmes to a client, with a key worker co-ordinating the client's participation and progress. One of these programmes may be counselling. How much should the key worker learn about the client's progress in counselling?*

Where do people get their information?

Knowledge is derived from a variety of sources and from critical comparison. It is not enough to say 'my neighbour said…' or 'my friend told me'. It can be asserted that people who undertake a university degree and those who use analysis in their work roles are trained to search for different sources of information, evaluate sources critically, and then develop their own views, based on the different sources of available evidence.

However, the skill of critical evaluation is not widespread. Many people live in communities of relatives and their wider extended family, that they turn to when they are in need of help. Michael Young and Peter Willmott studied this way of life in 1955 in *Family and Kinship in East London*, and commented that it was a way of life that was beginning to vanish. Subsequent reports over the years (Goodman, 2018; CPA, 2014) chart the decline of community ties as individuals leave their childhood communities for educational and employment opportunities, and the subsequent problems of caring for older people who have no relatives living nearby. However, a life lived in a community of relatives can sometimes seem too enclosed. There may be little tolerance of individual differences. Community members may gain their knowledge of the world primarily from each other – hearsay, gossip, 'common sense', clichés, and what 'they' say. These are their dominant sources of knowledge. Lack of critical thinking reinforces stereotypes and feeds unwitting prejudice, even when the community supports a sense of belonging.

> Practice Example 7.3 *A young man grew up in a community surrounded by his parents, aunts and uncles, brothers and sisters, cousins, and grandparents. At first he found this closeness reassuring, but as he began to grow up, he became aware that he was gay, and he did not dare to tell his family, because he had heard their hostile statements against homosexual people. He feared that if he told them about his sexuality, they would reject him. Eventually, his emotional despair and the strain of secrecy led to him leaving home and living many miles away, where he maintained little contact with his family. His family members were bewildered and hurt by his seeming rejection of them.*

As well as acquiring information from members of their communities, families, neighbours, and from formal education, individuals gather knowledge from the press, television, advertising, and from social media. But which information is trustworthy? Which information is believable? A critical sense of comparison and evaluation helps an individual unpick the grains of truth from different versions of the 'facts'.

> Practice example 7.4 *The 'telephone game', when played by children, illustrates how an identical story, repeated one by one from person to person in a queue, ends up being a different story when the end of the queue is reached. Repetition and verbal transmission from one individual to another changes the facts and meaning of a message.*

People may begin to feel confused about how they can recognise information that they can believe in and trust. Modern life bombards individuals with information, not all of it authentic. Clients, patients, and users of services who seek help from professional practitioners may feel troubled about what some other person – a partner, a neighbour, or a relative – has told them. They may all too easily believe that what they have been told is the 'truth'.

> Practice example 7.5 *A woman whose former partner had exerted excessive control over her felt emotionally shattered. Now, although she was separated from him, she was being told by 'friends' that*

he was currently informing others that she was 'no good'. She believed what the friends said and felt downcast and depressed, believing that others would accept this opinion of her. The counsellor asked if she trusted her friends. They were 'his' friends, she replied. The counsellor then asked 'why do you continue to listen to them and believe what they say?'

Therapeutic information-giving

Therapeutic information-giving will try to

- offer choices
- suggest alternative courses of action and sources of information
- explore different points of view
- avoid being directive or judgemental
- encourage trying a new idea or approach
- emphasise that the choice of action has to be the person's own decision
- build confidence to accept a new approach or belief
- reduce feelings about an assumed threat from daring to think differently

Practice Example 7.6 An activity centre located in an inner city area had successfully reached out to the local community, and now had several women who were service users serving as board members. I attended a board meeting as part of a research project. One of the agenda items was about planning an annual presentation to which members of the community would be invited. The staff reported with enthusiasm that they were receiving many RSVPs. I noticed that the service user board members made little comment and looked rather uneasy. After the board meeting I had a meeting scheduled with the service users. I asked them what they thought of the board meeting. After some hesitation, one of the service users asked 'What does RSVP stand for?' I explained that RSVP was a French phrase (respondez s'il vous plait – respond if you please) whose abbreviation is often used on invitations to inform the person who is invited to send a response indicating whether or not they will be attending. At the meeting, none of the service users who were present had sufficient confidence to admit that they did not know the meaning of the phrase, and let the moment pass without comment, although they were mystified and felt very insecure.

The democratising movement in health and social services

From the 1970s onwards, new kinds of communication with service users became popular as part of a democratising movement within health and social services. The democratising movement included recognition of service users' voices, the determination to tackle widespread poverty and inequality, and efforts to combat different kinds of inter-sectionality.

Learning new behaviour through receiving new information was now being offered as a non-stigmatising endeavour. The new approach of bringing about change by empowering individuals to gain new knowledge and skills contrasted with previously dominant therapeutic approaches that emphasised a psychoanalytic approach (Freud, 1986) delivered by authoritative therapists who interpreted clients' statements and non-verbal communications in seemingly mysterious and unfathomable ways. Mayer and Timms (1970, discussed also in Chapter 4) published their research findings of clients who sought help for practical problems of poverty and were instead were offered analytic therapy. The analytic approach began to fall from favour following the publication of Mayer and Timms' book. Services began to focus on combating poverty and addressing structural inequalities.

Providing information became part of a democratic strategy. Agencies provided explanatory leaflets for a range of helping organisations and conditions. Supportive groups offered helpful information. A new emphasis on joining together in an egalitarian way predominated. Interest groups, adult education groups, and children's centres flourished. The professional practitioners who traditionally staffed service organisations were joined by increasing numbers of para-professionals, who lacked a professional qualification but had previously experienced the same problems as people who use services. The para-professionals (Higham, 2006, p. 21) began to help deliver the new group programmes. As part of this changed approach, informal training programmes to develop the skills and knowledge of clients, service users and patients were established. The training did not require an assessment or a pass mark, but imparted an egalitarian spirit of building skills and confidence through information-giving.

Three programmes that use information-giving

This chapter will discuss three programmes, developed in the 1960s and 1970s, that use information-giving as a strategy: assertiveness training, parenting training, and children's centres.

Assertiveness training

Teaching people to practise assertive skills first became popular in the 1970s (Smith, 1975; Lindenfield, 1986). The idea took hold that assertiveness is a desirable trait that helps individuals initiate actions which are neither aggressive nor passive, but are assertive, thus enabling them to communicate effectively, especially when communicating with figures of authority in a range of real-life situations. Assertiveness training takes place in supportive groups that provide information about how individuals can learn to be assertive. The target groups for this training are professional practitioners, but also, and most importantly, users of services, patients, and clients.

The training typically covers the following information:

1. Definitions of assertiveness and its opposites, non-assertiveness (passivity) and aggressiveness.

Assertiveness means expressing personal thoughts, emotions, beliefs and opinions honestly and appropriately, with respect for the thoughts, feelings, opinions and beliefs of others.

Non-assertive responses are *aggressive or passive*. Aggressive responses include rushing someone unnecessarily, 'telling' rather than 'asking', ignoring someone, and not considering the other person's feelings. Passivity means a failure to communicate one's own thoughts or feelings or doing things you don't want to do to please others, and letting others take responsibility for making decisions.

2. Characteristics and causes of assertiveness, passivity, and aggression, and why assertiveness is a valuable trait.

Assertiveness is a balanced response that is neither passive nor aggressive, which encourages others to be open and honest about their views, wishes and feelings. Being assertive means listening to others' views and responding appropriately (whether you agree or not), expressing appreciation of what others do, admitting your own mistakes and apologising, and keeping self-control.

An individual who continually uses passivity and aggression to respond to social situations will magnify their own communication problems so that they become less successful in 'getting through' to others. The underlying causes of non-assertiveness and passive responses are usually lack of self-confidence, thinking of themselves as unequal to others, and a strong need to be liked. Continual passive responses diminish an individual's feelings of self-worth; responding in a passive or non-assertive manner implies compliance with others' wishes. Passive responses encourage reciprocal treatment that reinforces a passive role. Individuals with low self-esteem may unwittingly invite others to treat them in the same way. Low self-esteem is then reinforced in a circle of passivity and reduced self-confidence.

Responding aggressively undermines others' rights and self-esteem. An individual with good interpersonal skills is likely to be aware of the different ways that people communicate, and learn how to respond appropriately. Aggressive behaviour fails to consider the views or feelings of other individuals, and fails to praise or appreciate others' efforts. Aggressive responses will encourage another person to respond aggressively or passively. Manipulation of others can be a disguised form of aggression, whilst humour can also be used aggressively.

3. Communication strategies that build assertiveness

Sometimes people say 'yes' to requests when they actually want to say 'no'. Assertiveness means considering the request in the **light of the other tasks that need to be done, and giving a truthful, tactful polite response.** Assertiveness requires **co-operation and negotiation**. However, it is very important to remember that using assertiveness is inappropriate if the other person is behaving irrationally. You must not risk your safety nor put yourself in physical danger, so it is wise to exercise professional judgement if a risk of harm seems likely.

4. Exercises to practise assertive responses

Communication interactions are two-way processes, and recipients' reactions may vary. You can begin to build assertiveness and valuing others' contributions by using open questioning, using empathy, seeking others' opinions, and including colleagues in a group discussion; listening carefully to what others say; using appropriate non-verbal and verbal responses, polite questioning, reflecting, clarifying, summarising; and giving yourself time to think about an issue before giving a response.

Two techniques that can aid assertiveness are *fogging* and the *broken record*. Fogging involves building a verbal wall of 'fog' in response to others' aggression – offering a calm, brief, non-defensive response, and agreeing with any areas of truth in what the other person says rather than arguing or disagreeing. The intent is that your calmness and non-confrontational manner will cause the other person's aggression to fade away. The *broken record* technique involves repeating what you want, time and time again, without raising the tone of your voice, without becoming angry, and by remaining calm and focussed on what you want. Both techniques have to be used sensitively and with discretion to avoid causing unintentional harm. Other assertiveness techniques include strategies for dealing with criticism, giving and receiving compliments, and positive and negative enquiry.

Parenting skills programmes

Parenting skills programmes were developed as part of the democratisation of health and social services during the 1960s and 1970s. Their emergence was an acknowledgement that communities were changing, adult children often lived at a distance from their childhood homes, and when they became parents themselves were not always able to turn to their own parents for help and support because of the distance involved. Traditionally, a young mother turned to her own mother and grandmother for advice and practical help during a pregnancy and after the birth. Communication and knowledge remained in the family and the tight-knit community and was passed down through generations, but at the time of the Industrial Revolution and the growth of industry in the nineteenth century, families were uprooted from their rural surroundings. Concern began to be expressed at the poor health of mothers and children and the high rates of infant mortality. This concern led to the establishment of health visiting (first called 'sanitary visitors') as a professional role in the early twentieth century. One of health visiting's goals was to further maternity and infant and child welfare by providing health education and reaching out to infants, their families and communities. Gradually the work of health visitors extended from one-to-one contacts to group work and teaching (Adams, 2012).

Parenting programmes began in the 1960s–1970s as part of the democratising movement. The programmes provide new parents with group learning, support, information about different parenting styles, children's development stages, and problem solving, in the belief that parenting is a skill that is learned. Parenting classes were designed to build existing skills, rather than labelling individuals as 'good' or 'bad' parents. Asking for help is praised; attitudes are non-judgemental. Classes focus on providing education and advice on bringing up children, and sharing experiences without judgement. Since the 1970s, these courses have thrived.

One of the first popular parenting programmes was the psychologist Dr. Thomas Gordon's P.E.T (Parent Effectiveness Training), which was introduced in 1962 in the USA, but was widely used in the UK. Gordon taught communication skills and conflict resolution. Influenced by Carl Rogers (1961), his training programme included amongst its communication strategies active listening and 'no-lose' conflict resolution. He wrote *Parent Effectiveness Training* in 1970.

Another well-known parenting programme is Systematic Training for Effective Parenting (the STEP Programme) developed in the 1970s by Don Dinkmeyer and Gary McKay in the USA, but also widely used in the UK. Their *Parent's Handbook* is aimed at providing parents with knowledge about how to be confident in communicating with their children. STEP's seven session course is designed to improve communication with the family.

Topics include communicating with your child, handling naughty behaviour, encouraging child–parent communication, anticipating the consequences of actions, meeting together as a family, and preventing drug and alcohol misuse. The STEP programme promotes human dignity and mutual respect, and includes reflective listening and cooperation.

Dinkmeyer, McKay, and Gordon were influenced by the writings of Alfred Adler (Adler, 1925, 1929, translated by R. Radin). Adler was a Viennese psychoanalyst who broke away from Freud's circle and turned from analysis to develop a theoretical system of Individual Psychology that focussed on individuals within their social environments, an approach similar to those of Maslow (1954) and Bronfenbrenner (1979). Adler also developed the concept of the inferiority complex.

Children's centres

Children's centres were introduced in the USA as part of the US government's 'war on poverty' in the 1960s. The government set up centres known as 'Head Start' in 1965 to meet emotional, psychological health, nutritional, and social needs of children under five years old to help them be prepared for school. The programmes were particularly targeted at children in low income families. In the UK, Sure Start Centres were set up in 1998, and were patterned on the Head Start model. The Centres provide integrated early learning and child care, health programmes for infants, play sessions, family support, advice on parenting and local services, and ante and post natal support. The Centres provide optimistic, welcoming, accessible environments for families with babies and young children and were intended to be an asset to the communities in which they were located. The Centres were run as partnerships of health, education, parents, and charities, rather than by local authorities. Different evaluation strategies were utilised to show that Sure Start programmes were delivering effective outcomes, with the results not entirely conclusive in the first years.

Naomi Eisenstadt, who was the director of the Sure Start programme in its beginning years, told the story of how the Sure Start Programmes were set up as part of New Labour's policies, how the programmes changed over time because of changing government policies and practice, and perhaps a lack of consistent government support (Eisenstadt, 2011). Yet many centres have survived and continue their work, communicating well with parents, children, and the community.

> Practice Example 7.7 The Chilwell Sure Start Centre in Nottingham is located on a council estate next to a primary school, and is on a bus route and near the tram. The atmosphere created by the staff is friendly and welcoming. Mothers and children come to the Centre to have their babies weighed, for advice, and to take part in group sessions on different topics. The Centre runs play sessions for mothers and babies. Information leaflets on services in the community, benefits, and other activities are prominently displayed.

Summary

This chapter has portrayed the giving of information – not advice – as a communication strategy that can educate and support individuals and families to develop the skills to make more confident, better informed choices for themselves and their families. The growth of information-giving coincided with the democratisation of health and social services in the 1960s and 1970s, which led to the start up of informal educational programmes like assertiveness training, parenting skills training, and the establishment of children's centres. The examples I have given are strategies that were first introduced in the USA and then imported into the UK some time later. Although I have focussed in the examples on groups that provide information and informal training, information-giving is also a helpful communication strategy to bear in mind for one-to-one practice in health, social work, and counselling.

References

Adams, C. (2012) *The History of Health Visiting*, Institute of Health Visiting, London. https://ihv. org.uk/about us/history-of-health-visiting/a-paper-by-cheryll-adams/

Adler, Alfred (1925, 1929) *The Practice and Theory of Individual Psychology*, translated by P. Radin. Routledge: New York.

Bronfenbrenner, U. (1979) *The Ecology of Human Development*. Harvard University Press: Cambridge, MA.

CPA Centre for Policy on Aging (2014) *Review: Changing family structures and their impact on the care of older people*. CPA: London.

Dinkmeyer, D. Sr., McKay, Gary, and Dinkmeyer, D.Jr. (2008 edition), *The Parent's Handbook: Systematic Training for Effective Parenting*. STEP Publishers: Fredericksburg VA.

Eisenstadt, Naomi (2011) *Providing a Sure Start: How Government Discovered Early Childhood*. Policy Press: London.

Freud, S. (1986) *The Essentials of Psycho-Analysis, selected by Anna Freud*. Penguin: London.

Goodman, Peter S. (2018) In Britain, Austerity Is Changing Everything. *New York Times*, 28 May, New York.

Gordon, Thomas (1970, 2002) *Parent Effectiveness Training*. Random House: New York.

Higham, Patricia (2006) *Social Work. Introducing Professional Practice*. Sage: London.

Lindenfield, G. (1986) *Assert Yourself. How to re-programme your mind for positive action*. Thorsens Publishers Limited: Wellingborough.

MaslowA. H. (1954). *Motivation and Personality*. Harper and Row: New York

Mayer, J. E. and Timms, N. (1970) *The Client Speaks: Working class impressions of casework*. Atherton: Oxford.

Rogers, C. R. (1961) *On Becoming a Person*. Constable: London.

Smith, M. J. (1975) *When I Say No, I Feel Guilty*. Bantam Books: New York.

Young, M. and Willmott, P. (1955, 1992) *Family and Kinship in East London*. Penguin: London.

Chapter 8

Ethical concerns for communication and interviewing

Why ethical issues arise

Ethical concerns are major influences on communication and interviewing skills. Understanding of the complexity of ethical issues increases as perceptions of ourselves and our society become more searching. Ethical issues arise in professional practice because we are all flawed human beings. New ethical issues can challenge traditional methods of communication. For example, a practitioner may privately realise that he has begun to dislike a particular person who uses services, or, alternatively, may be aware of having strong positive feelings for them; or the professional relationship may lack trust on the part of either the practitioner or the user of services, or both. These uncomfortable feelings can be explored by reflecting on the ethical codes of each profession, and by thoughtful open discussion during professional supervision. The practitioner who is honest and open will be ready to look at 'self'. This is not easy because an internal gaze often becomes an uncomfortable exercise. Ethical behaviour demands personal honesty and self-scrutiny, and this can deplete the practitioner's energy and motivation. Every profession is damaged when some of its registrants fall short of the expected ethical standards. For example, some practitioners fail to turn up for appointments or may cause intentional harm by acting dishonestly, stealing money, falsifying travel claims, and writing bogus reports –behaviour that may result in them being struck from their professional register and losing their profession.

Practice is individual and idiosyncratic, and each new situation raises ethical issues. A practitioner's own point of view may become clouded and biased amidst the pressures of practice. To acquire an objective perspective of one's own practice, it is advisable to make use of professional supervision, continuing professional development, and self-reflection to avert potentially harmful, inappropriate decisions. Failure to maintain an appropriate level of expertise constitutes an ethical failing. Maintaining an acceptable standard of professional practice requires commitment – consistent efforts of self-reflection, learning from professional supervision and undertaking continuing professional development as well as acquiring appropriate experience.

Ethical concerns are triggered when a practitioner misuses their authority and power in professional relationships with a person who uses services. The choice of language (as discussed in Chapter 3) can become an ethical barrier to effective communication. Overuse of technical diagnostic language may result in ethically dubious labelling of the individual. Complex professional language, jargon, and acronyms impede the effectiveness of an interview with a person whose first language is not English, whose identity developed from a different culture, who has a disability, or who is emotionally devastated by life events.

Conflicts of Interest

Ethical issues include conflicts of interest (BASW, 2012, 2014; NASW, 2017; NCS, 2018; BACP, 2016). Conflicts of interest arise when the boundaries of professional relationships are breached inappropriately, for example, by turning the professional relationship into a personal friendship or by beginning a sexual relationship with a client (Bond, 2015, pp. 157–9). A conflict of interest occurs when the practitioner adopts an overly powerful and controlling relationship with the client (Bond, 2015, pp. 88–89). Breaches of confidentiality destroy the professional relationship and signify a lack of respect for the person who uses services. Potential pitfalls that threaten to sabotage professional communication may occur because of the practitioner's vulnerability to becoming over-involved or their lack of insight into their own motivations. It is all too easy for a beginning practitioner to unwittingly allow a defence mechanism (Freud, 2018, 1936) to distort a professional relationship, for example, *projection* (projecting uncomfortable emotions onto another person), *transference* (a feeling towards another person that is transferred from a previous relationship), and *counter-transference* (where the person who receives a transference transfers back a feeling from a previous relationship).

Practice example 8.1: A student began a placement in children's services. Her tutor was concerned that the student's practice might be damaged by memories of her previous experiences of domestic violence, and spoke to the student about this risk. The student acknowledged the risk, and during her placement supervision discussed her past history with insight, used supervision positively, and completed the placement with an excellent practice report.

Patients/service users/clients influence professional communication

Society's understanding of professional power is changing. The public's increasing disillusionment with governmental institutions, medicine, education, and other public services challenges the hegemony of professional power. Changed perceptions of power require practitioners to re-examine how they communicate with service users.

Practice Example 8.2 At a local authority children's centre that promoted the health and well-being of parents and children under five, parents who were board members expressed frustration about sharing their ideas with staff members, who were perceived as using the parents' ideas without acknowledgement or payment. The parent board members felt that parents who received benefits were exploited by staff who earned salaries. The staff drew on the knowledge of local parent leaders but apparently had not made an equitable exchange for the knowledge.

Question: What kinds of communication might have prevented the parents from feeling exploited?

Intersectionality changes the ways practitioners communicate

As discussed previously, *intersectionality* – the inter-connections between race, class, disability, gender, disadvantage, and stigma, etc. (Collins and Bilge, 2016) – may decrease a practitioner's confidence in their ability to communicate effectively. Alternatively, *intersectionality* can help practitioners acquire a more subtle understanding of the person who seeks help. It's not just a matter of grasping the impact of *one* set of practical and emotional issues that arise from *one* aspect of being perceived as 'different', it's the combined impacts of several perceived 'differences' that can overwhelm the individual and the practitioner, who may struggle to understand what is happening.

> Practice example 8.3: A 75-year-old widow faced the task of re-fashioning her life. She was troubled by grief but also by underlying feelings of being 'different'. She had experienced poverty, and the deaths of her parents and her infant child as well as the recent death of her husband. These memories came flooding back. She felt undervalued by society's perception of old age, noticing that many people expected her to be confused and incapable of managing her own affairs. She was urged to give up many of her activities now that she was old and alone, but what she wanted was to find something meaningful to do. These experiences and societal attitudes filled her memories and emotions at the time of her husband's death, but her feelings were more complex than mourning her most recent loss.
>
> Question: How would you, as a practitioner, communicate with this woman?

Recognising the complex intertwined nature of her inner concerns, and the *intersectionality* that influenced her emotions might help you offer a sensitive response. You need to consider a range of individuals whose lives are marked by complex intersectionality – think of refugees, victims of domestic violence, and individuals whose ethic identities have resulted in negative labelling. Understanding how identities and experiences affect well-being requires careful consideration of how *intersectionality* impacts on the life of a particular individual.

Information empowers but poses risks

Society's changing values challenge professional power. Increasingly, people live in a consumer society. The rights of the 'consumer', with increased access to internet information, also challenge traditional power structures.

> Question: Who are the consumers?

They are the users of public services. Some service users may perceive that continuing to receive services depends on their willingness to agree with the practitioner's recommendations, but others will have the courage to express their disagreements and mount challenges.

The growth of the internet has led to breaches of privacy and increased victimisation. New legal controls have been introduced. The General Data Protection Regulation (GDPR) (EU) 2016/679, which came into force in 2018, is a European regulation on data protection and privacy, including exporting outside the European Union (EU) and the European Economic Area (EEA). The GDPR gives EU citizens and residents more control over their personal data through new requirements on how personal data is recorded, how it is processed, who has access to it, how widely it can be disseminated, and how long it can be stored. For example, personal data must be stored in conditions of privacy, using pseudonyms or anonymised versions of people's personal data should not be publicly available without the person giving informed consent. Data breaches must be reported within a set timescale. Individuals have a right to request copies of their personal data, and if they wish, that it be destroyed. Organisations have to appoint a data protection officer (DPO) to manage their GDPR compliance. The UK gave royal assent to the Data Protection Act 2018, which has equivalent requirements to the European legislation.

The importance of professional judgement

Effective communication relies not only on technical mastery, but also on exercising sound *professional judgement*. Every practitioner finds it challenging to know how and when to reach a sound professional judgement on whether to intervene in situations that pose a danger to the self and/or to others, or when it is justified to break confidentiality and limit a person's privacy or freedom. Kettle (2018, p. 229) suggests that social workers engaged in child protection maintain a balancing act of knowledge, skills, intuition, practice, tenacity, and courage to deal with different possibilities and explanations. They must be able to recognise when that balance is lost; their organisations need to support them in maintaining the balance; and professional training and practice should keep the child as the centre of concern, but take account of the complex contexts that surround the child.

When problems are complex and linked to ethical concerns, it may be necessary to refer a person to more specialist expertise. A relatively inexperienced practitioner may find it difficult to make effective judgements about when to refer a client/service user to specialist expertise. Working beyond the limit of one's competence by disregarding signs of a person's vulnerability can exacerbate stress and anxiety, and fail the person both ethically and therapeutically.

Professional judgement develops from a process of two-way communication, where you, the practitioner, communicate with the person who seeks your help, and where that person communicates their needs to you. You need to encourage the participation of the person seeking help, and listen carefully. Sometimes loyalty to one's employer can overwhelm niggles of doubt and uncertainty that every practitioner feels at times. Are you meant to enforce the rules of the organisation above all else? Suppose you inadvertently discover that injustices have occurred, albeit unintentionally? Your professional judgement may be difficult to determine and then act upon. Professional supervision can help a practitioner maintain objectivity and engage ethically with clients.

For counsellors in private practice, professional judgement includes considering the ethics of charging fees in private practice.

Questions: What about the client who cannot afford to pay? Suppose a client with ample finances whose psychological state has improved after twelve weeks of counselling asks you to continue the weekly contact? Would the thought of earning more money sway the counsellor to say yes?

Shared confidentiality

A key issue is the growing complexity of maintaining confidentiality. Instead of absolute confidentiality, a practitioner nowadays must take note of legal requirements to protect individuals from harm, and that includes reporting instances of suspected abuse and situations when the practitioner's own safety and/or the service user's safety may be at risk: These exceptions to absolute confidentiality should be explained to the client/user of services at the beginning of professional contacts.

The BACP Framework of Ethics (2018) aims to protect confidentiality, inter alia, by

- *actively protecting information about clients from unauthorised access or disclosure*
- *informing clients about how personal data and information will be used and who is within the circle of confidentiality*
- *requiring that all recipients of personally identifiable information treat such information as confidential*
- *informing clients about any reasonably foreseeable limitations of privacy or confidentiality, for example in supervision or protecting a client or others from serious harm*

The *circle of confidentiality* mentioned by the BACP Framework is a concept that needs more scrutiny. I consider the 'circle' to be one way of describing *shared confidentiality*.

Question: What is *shared confidentiality?*

Shared confidentiality describes how information may be shared within an organisation. The professional practitioner who practises in an organisation with other professional practitioners and support staff may set limits on how much of the client's information should be divulged to colleagues, but in reality, some measure of confidentiality is shared, to some extent, within an office – telephone calls, messages, holiday cover, and emergencies require some sharing of information about the client. The concept of *shared confidentiality* needs to be further explored, particularly now that GDPR regulations are in force, to ensure that the spirit of the regulations is upheld, and that practitioners are clear about the limits and extent of *shared confidentiality*. Shared confidentiality should not mean sharing every detail about a client.

Codes of ethics are changing in response to public concerns

A professional code helps to remind a practitioner of their profession's required ethical behaviour, and also spells out the penalties of breaching the code, such as suspension from practice, or removal from registration (being struck off). Social workers, counsellors, and health practitioners want their professional practice to adhere to ethical codes. Not doing so risks the possibly of de-registration and loss of one's professional role. Self-interest and self-protection motivate practitioners to profess their commitment to professional values. But their motivation is also altruistic, and propels them towards strong commitments to ethical codes designed to protect the public.

Commonalities and differences in ethical codes

Codes of ethics contain detailed ethical principles, with a synergy between them, but also differences. Each profession's ethical statement explains their understanding of their profession's values, for example, maintaining confidentiality, protecting data, safeguarding vulnerable people from harm, and ensuring that registered professional practitioners practise within the limits of their competence. Ethical codes are living documents that continually need updating in response to new ethical issues.

The biomedical code of ethics is based on four principles: beneficence (doing good); non-maleficence (doing no harm); respect for autonomy and truth; and justice (Eby, 2000). An important ethical principle of every profession is to 'do no harm'. An initial contact stage provides a practitioner with opportunities to undertake a 'risk of harm' analysis to protect a service user or patient or client from harm. Neglecting the therapeutic imperative to 'do no harm' constitutes an ethical and therapeutic failure. Choosing appropriate communication techniques and using them with skill and insight can help clients modify their thinking and emotions, and abate their perceived problems. The Nolan Principles (Committee on Standards in Public Life, 1995) provide ethical guidance to holders of public office, and are used widely in the health service. The seven Principles are: (1) selflessness, (2) integrity, (3) objectivity, (4) accountability, (5) openness, (6) honesty, and (7) leadership.

Ethical codes for counselling focus on ethical concerns within therapeutic relationships. Social work codes include the expectations that social workers will be activists who seek to change unjust systems and help disadvantaged people. The codes draw on common law, legal statutes, and accepted principles of justice and fairness derived from philosophy and major religions. Ethical codes are characterised by growing complexity, as they take account of new technologies, new definitions of equality, and a broader range of concerns.

Ethical codes become more complex as public awareness of previously unacknowledged inequalities and injustices grows, and as legislation expands. Views and attitudes about inequalities, both positive and negative, may seem entrenched amongst certain populations, but are changing in other populations. Ethical codes' expansion of detail, scope, and range of coverage pose a risk that practitioners might perceive the codes as overly-long detailed lists of prohibitions for practice. Practitioners should be familiar with the key ethical principles that comprise the substance of a code, and use this as their guide for effective communication and interviewing.

Ethical codes for counselling

Two examples of counselling ethical codes share some similarities, but differ in what they identify and how they communicate their understanding of the implications of a Code.

Table 8.1 Two ethical codes for counselling

BACP Ethical Framework for the Counselling Professions (BACP, 2018, accessed 5 July 2018)	*National Counselling Society Code of Ethics (accessed 5 July 2018)*
Principles of being trustworthy, autonomy, beneficence, non-maleficence (doing no harm), justice, and self-respect.	Principles of working towards the good of clients and doing no harm (beneficence and non-maleficence); being trustworthy and responsible (fidelity); respect for the dignity and rights of the client (autonomy); justice; and integrity and self-responsibility.
Good practice expectations of putting clients first; working to professional standards; showing respect; building an appropriate relationship with clients; breaks and endings; integrity; accountability and candour; confidentiality; working with colleagues and in teams; supervision; training and education; trainees; research; care of self as a practitioner; and responding to ethical dilemmas and issues.	Offering and delivering a service; advertising, display of credentials and use of titles, confidentiality, maintenance of records and recording of sessions; continuing professional development (CPD) and supervision; treatment of minors and those classified as persons with special needs or vulnerabilities.
Values include respecting human rights and dignity; alleviating symptoms of personal distress and suffering; enhancing people's well-being and capability; improving the quality of relationships between people; increasing personal resilience and effectiveness; facilitating a sense of self meaningful to the person(s) concerned within their personal and cultural context; appreciating the variety of human experience and culture; protecting clients' safety; ensuring the integrity of practitioner–client relationships; enhancing the quality of professional knowledge and its application; and striving for the fair and adequate provision of services.	Requirements for general conduct, training ethics, relationship with the society, and a prohibition on use of conversion (reparative) therapy, e.g. the counsellor must not offer counselling that offers sexual orientation change efforts or seeks to eliminate or reduce same sex attraction in clients; and guidance on communications and social media.

Source: Websites of the British Association of Counselling and Psychotherapy, and the National Counselling Society

Social work codes of ethics

UK and US social work codes differ but share some similarities.

Communication and confidentiality in research

Social and psychological research involves people as research participants. In the past, individuals were not always informed about the nature of a particular piece of research and the reasons why it was being conducted. They were kept in ignorance. Researchers were powerful authority figures, who too often did not consider it necessary to be open and honest with the people they were researching. This attitude has now changed, and the public reacts in horror to past actions that disregarded people's rights.

Practice example 8.4: *In previous generations, incoming students at Wellesley College and similar 'Ivy League' colleges in the USA were required to have a 'posture picture' taken. Photographs of each individual student standing in their underclothes were taken from the front, back, and side view, ostensibly to examine the student's posture. In the 1990s, the posture pictures were discovered to be covert research on body types by the Harvard University psychologist William Sheldon. The students had never been told the true purpose of the pictures, and their consent to participate in the research had not been obtained.*

Table 8.2 Placeholder text as need caption and source Two ethical codes for social work

British Association of Social Workers Code (2012, 2014)	*National Association of Social Workers (USA) Code (1996, 2008)*
Values and ethical principles of upholding and promoting human dignity and well-being; respecting the right to self-determination; promoting the right to participation; treating each person as a whole person; identifying and developing strengths of individuals; challenging discrimination, recognising diversity; upholding the values and reputation of the profession; being trustworthy; maintaining professional boundaries; making considered professional judgements; and being professionally accountable.	Responsibilities for maintaining the profession's integrity and for avoiding actions that may breach ethical standards: that practitioners should be honest, seek help for any of their own problems that might affect professional judgement, avoid misrepresentations of facts and policies, and acknowledge contributions made by others.
Developing professional relationships, assessing and managing risk, acting with the informed consent of service users, unless required by law to protect that person or another from risk of serious harm, providing information, using authority in accordance with human rights principles, empowering people, challenging the abuse of human rights, being prepared to whistleblow, maintaining confidentiality, maintaining clear and accurate records, striving for objectivity and self-awareness in professional practice, using professional supervision and peer support to reflect on and improve practice, taking responsibility for their own practice and continuing professional development, contributing to the continuous improvement of professional practice, taking responsibility for the professional development of others, and facilitating and contributing to evaluation and research.	Responsibilities for developing appropriate skills for supervision and consultation, evaluating performance effectively, avoiding exploitation of supervisees/students, maintaining and storing accurate and confidential records in accordance with required statutes and contracts, observing ethical protocols when transferring clients to other service provision, and advocating for adequate resources for services, and allocating resources fairly.
	Responsible to society as a whole for promoting general welfare and public participation, including assisting in public emergencies, and engaging in social and political action. Practitioners who are involved in organised labour union action should be guided by the profession's ethical standards. Practitioners should bill clients accurately, and not solicit referrals and testimonials.

Source: Websites of the National Association of Social Workers and the British Association of Social Workers

I discovered years later that as a young undergraduate, I had been one of the participants in this research at Wellesley College. At the time, I was a trusting young undergraduate believing that the staff had our best interests at heart. Years later, I was forced to rethink my previous assumptions.

In 2018, the British Association of Counselling and Psychotherapy (BACP) published new *Ethical Guidelines for Research in the Counselling Professions* (BACP, 2018). These guidelines, inter alia, remind practitioners of the importance of maintaining trust and trustworthiness, establishing an ethical relationship between the researcher and the participants, exercising social responsibility and working within the law, data protection, avoiding deception, awareness of a power balance, and the vulnerability of research participants. The Guidelines clearly seek to ensure that the deception and powerlessness of the research participants in the example discussed above should not take place within contemporary practice.

Personhood and non-judgemental attitudes

Maintaining non-judgemental attitudes does not mean confronting a person with one's own attitudes, but enabling the person to begin to consider their own attitudes. Practitioners should accept the individual's personhood (Rogers, 1951), and encourage users of services to examine their own attitudes and beliefs.

> Practice example 8.5 *A person with HIV confided his anger and disillusionment with the medication the doctor has prescribed, saying he wanted to rid his body of harmful substances. The counsellor began to suspect that the client had stopped taking the medication that prevented him from developing AIDS. Yet if the counsellor 'ordered' him to take the medication, as the doctor had done, the counsellor had no doubt that the client would immediately cease contact. The public health manager at the counselling organisation agreed that the client was putting himself at risk of AIDS because of failure to take his medication, but decided that because the client was not mentally disturbed, he had a right to make that decision.*

> *Question:* What are the ethical issues in this practice example?

Key issues for ethical communication

The key issues for maintaining ethical communication include:

- *do no harm*
- '*less is more*' (don't dominate the conversation)
- maintain *respect* for an individual's personhood
- *be honest*
- maintain *confidentiality* and *integrity*
- ensure that as a practitioner, you receive appropriate *professional supervision, support* and undertake *professional development*

The danger of working to ethical codes is that they can provide a false sense of security for the practitioner, and may dull the practitioner's ability to develop a deep awareness of the complex nature of communication. Willingness to engage and grapple sensitively with the ethical dilemmas of communication should be a requisite for all practitioners.

Summary: Demonstrating professional values in communication with service users

Codes and frameworks specify the ethical requirements of each profession, and shape the use of communication skills, but the codes do not provide a formula for responding to every ethical situation that arises in individual practice. The codes provide meaningful guidelines, but the practitioner has to think, reflect, and draw on their professional values. Effective communication skills are built on a foundation of values that are carefully considered.

I have identified four principles (Higham, 2006) that support and enable good communication.

- *The reciprocal influence of the environment on the individual, and the individual on the environment*
  This principle reminds practitioners to understand present happenings within a context of change, to acknowledge new concerns and recognise significant past events.
- *Change and development throughout human life*
  This principle reminds practitioners to acknowledge the complex, multi-layered nature of social and personal contexts that shape peoples' lives.
- *The intrinsic worth of an individual*
  This principle reminds practitioners to listen to the needs and wishes of people who use services and their carers, respond appropriately, and communicate with respect.
- *Empowerment*
  This principle reminds practitioners to practise in partnership with clients/patients/people who use services, build and promote their strengths.

References

BACP British Association of Counselling and Psychotherapy (2016) *Ethical Framework for the Counselling Professions*. BACP: Lutterworth.

BACP British Association of Counselling and Psychotherapy (2018) *Ethical Guidelines for Research in the Counselling Professions*. BACP: Lutterworth.

BASW British Association of Social Workers (2012, 2014) *Code of Ethics for Social Workers*. BASW: Birmingham.

Bond, T. (2015) *Standards and Ethics for Counselling in Action*. 4th Edition. Sage: London.

Collins, Patricia Hill, and Bilge, Sirma (2016) *Intersectionality*. Polity Press: Cambridge.

Committee on Standards in Public Life (1995) *Nolan Principles of Public Life* (Committee Website accessed 5 June 2018).

Eby, Maureen (2000) Chapter Six 'Producing evidence ethically' in Roger Gomm and Celia Davies (eds.), *Using Evidence in Health and Social Care*. Open University/Sage: London, pp. 108–128.

Freud, A. (2018, 1936) *The Ego and the Mechanisms of Defense*. Routledge: Abingdon.

GDPR (2016) The General Data Protection Regulation (GDPR) (EU) 2016/679https://eur-lex.europa.eu/eli/reg/2016/679/oj. Website accessed 9 December 2018.

Harari, Yuval Noah (2017) *Homo Deus: A Brief History of Tomorrow*. Vintage: London.

Higham, P. (2006) *Social Work: Introducing Professional Practice*. Sage: London.

Hood, Rick (2018) *Complexity in Social Work*. Sage: London.

Kettle, M. (2018) 'A balancing act: a grounded theory study of the professional judgement of child protection social workers' *Journal of Social Work Practice*. Volume 32, 2 June. pp. 219–231.

NASW (2017, 2008, 1996) NASW National Association of Social Workers (USA) Code of Ethics (Approved by the 2017 NASW Delegate Assembly) NASW: Washington DC.

NCS National Counselling Society (2018) *Code of Ethics*https://www.nationalcounsellingsociety. org/about-us/code-of-ethics/ accessed 8 December 2018.

Rogers, C. (1951) *Client-Centered Therapy: Its Current Practice, Implications and Theory*. Constable: London.

Wastell, D. and White, S. (2010) 'Technology as magic: Fetish and folly in the IT-enabled reform of children's services'. In Ayre, P. and Preston-Shoot, M. (eds), *Children's Services at the Crossroads: a Critical Evaluation of Contemporary Policy for Practice*. Russell House Publishing: Lyme Regis.

Chapter 9

Communication and interviewing in different organisational contexts

Communicating across professional boundaries

Professional practitioners in local authorities, voluntary and charitable organisations, educational institutions, health care organisations, private organisations, and practitioners in private practice use communication and interviewing skills as essential tools to shape their practice. Yet they may use these skills differently depending on their organisation's purpose.

Communicating across the professional boundaries of separate professions is now a necessary requirement of multi-professional practice. A professional practitioner's perspective of other professions and roles can be narrow – for example, social workers claiming to 'own' the 'social model' of intervention and defining the 'medical model' negatively.

> *Question:* Is it possible for members of separate professions to value each other's contributions, or will they doubt the value of working with other professions?

Organisational structures

Organisations design their structures to make it possible for them to achieve their aims and purposes. Because aims and purposes differ from one organisation to another, practitioners in a particular organisation use communication and interviewing skills in ways that may differ from other organisations. For example, professional practitioners in the National Health Service typically use interviewing skills as part of triage and diagnosis; social workers in local authorities use interviewing skills to assess needs and investigate safeguarding issues; counsellors in private practice interview clients to assess a client's mental and emotional health before beginning counselling.

Professional practitioners use communication skills for interviewing and gathering information, but also for building and sustaining relationships, and offering therapeutic support. Different professional training courses all teach communication and interviewing skills, suggesting a certain commonality of skills across the professions. However, problems may arise when practitioners have to communicate across organisational boundaries. Their internal systems of communication may function well, but might be less than effective for inter-professional communication. The use of unfamiliar jargon and acronyms can be alienating when used for inter-professional communication. Attitudes towards other professions may be based on negative stereotypes (as noted), and further impede communication.

As discussed in Chapter 3, social workers may perceive that they are practising a *social model* (Oliver, 1996) that encourages service users' voice to give their feedback about how services have been delivered. They may believe that health professionals will inevitably practice a *medical model*, in which professional power dominates and service users lack a voice. Social workers may believe (perhaps unconsciously) that social work has an exclusive ownership of the social model, and this mistaken belief may damage social workers' perceptions of health practitioners and lead to a lack of trust that sabotages inter-professional communication. Social workers hopefully will begin to acknowledge current changes in health care practice that seek to move practice away from an authoritarian paternalistic *medical model* towards more participatory *social models*.

The health professions continue to experience changes in how they deliver services, and how they communicate with their patients. Modern health care was built initially on authoritative disciplined regimes developed to prevent infection and epidemics – a real threat because, until relatively recently (within living memory), there were no antibiotics to fight infection. The influence of patient groups who provide feedback and new requirements for registration and re-registration of physicians have modified the traditional power structures. These developments have changed the way health professionals communicate with each other and with patients.

Counsellors may believe that they 'own' counselling skills, and perceive other professions as borrowing from counselling. This perception is mistaken. Health practitioners and social workers use counselling skills when communicating with patients and service users, and have done so for years. Social work, in particular, practised psycho–social case work (Hollis, 1972, 1964), which drew heavily on Freudian concepts as its dominant mode of intervention until the 1970s. Significantly, Mary Woods updated Hollis' methods and developed them further (Wood and Hollis, 1999) for contemporary practitioners. In an updated version of Hollis' book that conceptualised social work as a psycho–social process, Woods successfully blended Hollis' ideas with Bronfenbrenner's ecological theory that Germain and Gitterman later developed for social work practice (2008). Bond (2015, p. 27) acknowledges that counselling skills are used by other professions, but argues that the way these skills are articulated within counselling practice is helpful to other professional roles.

When professional practitioners begin to work in multi-professional teams, they may at first be surprised to discover commonalities of approach in the ways professional practitioners communicate with service users, patients, and clients. Professional training programmes cover similar ground in teaching practitioners how to use communication and interviewing skills. An individual profession does not 'own' these skills. Some practitioners may begin to feel deskilled, and wonder what their own contribution should be. Perhaps they might doubt the distinctiveness of their own profession. These feelings are understandable, and are heightened by frequent use of impenetrable jargon and acronyms.

Practice example 9.1 *Whilst serving as a lay member of an NHS organisation, I regularly received a thick bundle of papers to read in preparation for board meetings. I read the reports and minutes sitting at my computer, and frequently had to refer to the internet to help me decipher the meaning of the jargon and acronyms. I reflected that professional communication functions like a club that excludes the public from understanding.*

Multi-professional practice

Each profession can claim to be unique with its own particular knowledge, training, roles, identity, and skills, but some skills – particularly communication skills – are shared across the professions. All practitioners learn about communication skills and are expected to relate to people in a skilled manner, guided by their profession's ethical codes. Membership of a multi-professional team can raise issues about how communication is transacted between the different professional practitioners who are team members and how effective it is. An *authoritarian* model and a *medical model* may predominate. Some professions may feel threatened by the apparent confidence of other professions. There is a danger of competition rather than co-operation. Working in a multi-professional team can unwittingly lead to internal questioning about the value and uniqueness of one's own profession. Some new multi-professional structures try to overcome these barriers to collaboration.

Practice Example 9.2 Focus Independent Adult Social Work within North East Lincolnshire is a social enterprise, known as a social work practice, commissioned by the local NHS Clinical Commissioning Group (CCG) and the local authority, North East Lincolnshire Council. Focus has had the opportunity to develop a multi-professional model of communication: it is organised into teams of social workers and health professionals that provide complex case management to older people (including those with a mental health issue) and to adults with physical, sensory or learning disabilities; a service that provides the gateway to adult social work/care; an adult safeguarding team; a continuing care NHS healthcare team; and all support functions, including community care finance. Focus works collaboratively with another not-for-profit community interest company, NAViGO, which emerged from the NHS to run all local mental health and associated services. Focus also works closely with community organisations.

This practice example illustrates that multi-professional practice can become a reality if strategic planning by employers acknowledges its importance. In a multi-professional organisation, practitioners from different professions have to communicate with each other across agency boundaries. They have to become aware of different organisational aims and requirements, and take account of opportunities and disappointments posed by working alongside a different practice culture. They may feel challenged, deskilled, or misunderstood. The key to working together is to focus on the needs of the persons they are trying to help, and be confident of the value of their own contributions.

Organisational size

Professional practitioners work in large, medium-sized and small organisations or as independent practitioners. For example, counsellors are employed in private practice, or increasingly in the NHS to deliver the IAPT programme (Improved Access to Psychological Therapies). Local authorities and national charities employ the majority of social workers. Health professionals mainly work in the National Health Service in hospitals, specialist services, or in GP surgeries. In a large national organisation like the NHS, structures are complex. The NHS operates with devolved structures and delegated authority, but within a national remit of overall policy control. Local authorities deliver social services through devolved systems within internal organisational structures. Internal communication has a challenging remit to ensure that every practitioner obtains up-to-date information necessary for them to perform their professional roles.

Organisational systems for recording data

Organisations use complex systems to communicate and record data, and demonstrate objectivity and accountability. These complex communication systems may result in problems of excessive bureaucracy, lack of individual personal attention, and mistakenly treating all people the same rather than recognising their individuality. Organisational systems and procedures may trigger rigid, inflexible responses to people in need.

Organisations and bureaucracy

All organisations are bureaucracies with set procedures. Historically, the purpose of a 'bureaucracy' (Weber, 2009) was to provide honest, fair services and avoid corruption and favouritism. 'Bureaucracy' was viewed at first as a progressive concept, but contemporary society is more critical, recognising bureaucracies' tendency to develop intractable routines that submerge individual needs within inflexible policies and routines. Bureaucracies need to be tempered with humanity. This action does not begin or end with professional practitioners, but applies also to front-line administrative staff who answer telephones, staff front desks, and provide information to members of the public. Their contributions are vital to good communication, but sometimes can do damage if they function in rigid inflexible ways and treat people as objects.

> Practice example 9.3: *An information technology specialist in an engineering firm contracted a life threatening disease and died suddenly. Her husband telephoned the firm where she was employed to inform them of her death. He was put on hold for five minutes by the receptionist, then the receptionist came back on the line to say: 'I spoke to HR (human relations) and they say you must put it in writing.' The husband felt demeaned by the firm's bureaucratic manner. He reflected afterwards that the human relations department could have been more responsive and sensitive, but instead they delegated their response to the receptionist and, perhaps unwittingly, encouraged her to give a technically correct but bureaucratic response, without encouraging the expression of human concern.*

Why are procedures so often rigid? Why does communication sometimes disregard humanity? In contemporary society, organisations increasingly live in fear of data protection breaches, or failing to report safeguarding concerns, terrorist threats, and other violent incidents. To respond to these difficult situations, organisations develop bureaucratic procedures and train their staff accordingly. In atmospheres where fear and suspicion dominate, humanity may be pushed to one side. It takes an experienced practitioner to decide when a rigid protocol needs to be tempered with humanity, and when a sensitive human communication is the right response.

> Practice Example 9.4: *The widow of a retired man who had received a regular pension from his employer's pension fund informed the fund of her husband's death. She subsequently applied to her*

> husband's pension fund for a survivor's pension, to which she was entitled. She spoke on the telephone to a helpful member of staff who emailed clear information about how to apply for a survivor pension. She applied by post, but whilst waiting for a response, noted that the pension fund continued to post her husband's monthly pension cheque. She returned the first cheque to the pension fund with a letter explaining his death, but the next month, another cheque arrived in her husband's name. Then she received a stern letter from the chief executive officer of the pension fund, demanding that she return the overpayment. She felt confused and upset by the tone of this letter, which did not acknowledge that she had already returned one cheque and had applied to them for a widow's pension.

This practice example illustrates a lack of communication between different parts of an organisation. One part of the organisation helped the widow to obtain a survivor's pension; the other part threatened the widow to return the over-payment of the dead husband's pension. The organisation apparently failed to note the previous information from the widow that the pension recipient had died. A lack of internal communication overwhelmed the effectiveness of their operations and resulted in a lack of humanity.

Hood (2018) presents a comprehensive overview of management systems, including bureaucracy, 'command and control' management, motivation strategies, functions and processes, and performance management. He advocates using systems theory, drawing on the thinking of Bronfenbrenner's ecological systems (1979), Gitterman and Germain's environmental context systems (2008), Pincus and Minahan's helping systems (1973), and Minuchin's family systems (2012, 1974) to develop socio-technical systems that can help to overcome the 'control problem' and allow practitioners to become more responsive to people who need services. Although generally positive about systems, Hood (2018, p. 6) critiques systems theories' assumptions of being able to reach an end point of equilibrium and stability, commenting that systems theories may fail to explain the phenomena of creativity and innovation.

Sometimes the automated systems that organisations set up for communication convey a 'don't care' message to the public.

> Practice example 9.5 Lecturing staff at a large university could be reached on the telephone via their own individual extension number on the university switchboard. The lecturers were often away from their desks when they were teaching students. Their voice mails and automated email responses were not regularly updated. When their phone rang, and they did not reply, the caller was greeted by an automated statement, asking the caller to leave a message. One caller finally managed to reach a lecturer, after trying many extension numbers for other lecturers, and said, with an ironic sigh, 'at last, a human voice!'

This complex system of leaving messages effectively distanced the students from the lecturers. Complex systems create problems for achieving effective communication. The large size of organisational structures makes grasping the 'whole' of an organisation more and more difficult for practitioners, administrative staff members, and managers.

Small organisations are also not immune to internal communication breakdowns.

Practice example 9.6 *A small local charity which provided services to women seeking to rebuild their lives employed part time staff, used volunteers, and was governed by a board of voluntary trustees. When external damage occurred to their rented premises, threatening the safety of the building, the board initially struggled to communicate information and give their responses to the crisis to all the staff (who worked part time), the part time volunteers, and the clients so that they all understood what had happened.*

The board members used the occasion to review and improve their communication processes, recognising the challenges of conveying information efficiently to part time staff and volunteers. They identified the importance of delivering a clear full response to a crisis situation rather than partial statements to a few staff. The board's communication improved following this incident.

Personalisation makes new demands of professional communication

Leadbeater (2004) defined *personalisation* as giving people who use services more say in running services, deciding how money is spent on services, and providing opportunities to become co-designers and service producers. *Personalisation* developed as a different method of service delivery in adult social care, in contrast to large-scale bureaucracies delivering standardised services. Instead of institutionalised responses, *personalisation* tries to provide services tailored to individual wants and needs, for example, self-directed support and personal budgets that enable individuals who receive services to choose the help they want and need. The success of personalisation policy depends, inter alia, on good quality communication – providing accurate full information, advice, and advocacy that help service users choose what help they receive. Communication between the professional practitioner and the person requesting services becomes very different when the person begins to behave more like a 'customer'.

Two issues that threaten to sabotage the concept of personalisation are first, frequent organisational changes that delay service delivery; and second, insufficient staff and resources to deliver an effective personalised service. The service user is not always made aware of these issues when applying for a service.

Practice example 9.7 *McPherson (September 2018) recounts the frustrations he encountered when he tried to arrange social care support for his mother-in-law. He encountered poor communication throughout. Three social workers each conducted an initial assessment of needs, but his mother-in-law was not allocated a named social worker for ongoing contact. Later, a gap in care occurred when an NHS service withdrew and the local authority organised another service to deliver services in its place. During this period, his relative was left with no support for a week. When he tried to contact a social worker, he had to phone a call centre, and found that he was made to repeat the problem several times. Some social workers that he spoke to refused to provide their contact numbers because they only undertook assessments. There were frequent mistakes with the care package – carers came on the wrong days, and at the wrong times. At the time he wrote about his difficulties, his mother-in-law still had not been allocated a social worker, so it was difficult to know whom to contact when her problems continued to cause concern. He formed the impression that the family was being passed around from one service to another, with no clear explanation given. The standard of communication was poor.*

> *Question:* What kind of organisational communication systems might have helped to avoid this situation?

Summary

Organisational contexts are changing their expectations of how practitioners should communicate with clients, service users, and patients. Practitioners increasingly are expected to communicate with respect, to offer consultation, and to work in partnership, rather than with overt power and authority. The trend towards multi-professional practice places demands on practitioners. Keeping a collaborative focus on the needs of service users/clients/patients is to be desired, rather than allowing impersonal, bureaucratic, automated systems to dominate. Systems theories may provide strategies for encouraging non-bureaucratic professional communication. Individual practitioners may sustain a sense of purpose by participating in professional support groups that work for change.

References

Bond, T. (2015) *Standards and Ethics for Counselling in Action*. 4th Edition. Sage: London.

Bronfenbrenner, U. (1979) *The Ecology of Human Development*. Harvard University Press: Cambridge, MA.

Germain, C. and Gitterman, A. (2008) *The Life Model of Social Work Practice*. Columbia University Press: New York.

Hollis, F. (1972 edition, 1964) *Casework: A Psychosocial therapy*. 2nd edition revised. Random House: New York.

Hood, Rick (2018) *Complexity in Social Work*. Sage: London.

Leadbeater, C. (2004) *A summary of 'Personalisation through participation: a new script for public services.* Demos: London.

McPherson, Blair (2018) 'Dropping the ball – how one ex-social worker found the experience of arranging care for an elderly relative' http://www.communitycare.co.uk/2018/09/05/dropping-ball-one-ex-social-worker-found-experience-arranging-care-elderly-relative/ Website accessed 6 September 2018.

Minuchin, S. (2012, 1974) *Families and Family Therapy*. Harvard University Press: Cambridge MA.

Oliver, M. (1996) *Understanding Disability: From Theory to Practice*. Macmillan: Baskingstoke.

Pincus, A. and Minahan, A. (1973) *Social Work Practice: Model and Method*. Peacock: Itasca, IL.

Weber, Max (2009) *From Max Weber: Essays in Sociology*. edited by H.H. Gerth and C. Wright Mills, with Preface by Bryan S. Turner, pp. 196–244. Routledge: London.

Wood, Mary E. and Hollis, F. (1999) *Casework A Psychosocial Therapy*. 5th Edition. McGraw Hill: New York.

Chapter 10

Issues of communicating with technology, computers, and artificial intelligence

Development of technologies

Artificial intelligence and algorithms are significant contemporary developments of technology that influence human communication for better and, perhaps, for worse. Technology provides useful tools that can make life easier and more productive. This is not a new phenomenon. For example, invention of the wheel represented a growth in technology that enabled the development of travel and more efficient food production. A portrayal of nineteenth-century technology is found in Gore Vidal's novel, *Lincoln* (1984), about the life of the US President during the early 1860s. The novel provided details of how Lincoln used the modern technology of that era: the telegraph for sending messages to Union Army generals during the Civil War and for receiving messages so that he could discover in a relatively short time whether he had been re-elected as president; how he used steam boats to travel; and the railway to take him from Washington DC to the Pennsylvania battlefield where he delivered the Gettysburg address. Lincoln also used photography to establish his identity throughout the country when he ran for re-election. Steven Spielberg's 2012 film *Lincoln*, based on Doris Kearns Goodwin's 2005 book, *Team of Rivals: The Political Genius of Abraham Lincoln,* charted this use of technology in the events of Lincoln's life.

Successive generations have grown used to the introduction of new technologies that result in products that change the patterns of their lives, including invention of electricity, telephones, washing machines, vacuum cleaners, radio and television, motor cars, airplanes, tanks, dynamite, nuclear weapons and space travel. These inventions serve different purposes – some as weapons of war and destruction; some as appliances that make family life easier and more enjoyable, and some enhance the ways people communicate with each other. Questions have been asked recently about whether technological innovations serve purposes determined by human beings and whether human beings are in control of the technology. Professional practitioners will be aware of the advantages of using technology, both for professional and for private use, but also observe how some service users become addicted to social media and other technology, and seemingly replace human relationships in their lives. The chapter presents an overview of the development of technology in our lives, and explores some of the ethical issues that are raised about their use.

The use of computers

Computers are essential parts of contemporary communication systems, but the concept of 'computers' – machines that can be programmed to automatically 'compute' and carry out systematic operations – is not new. Charles Babbage, with Ada Lovelace, developed a primitive mechanical computer in early nineteenth-century England, representing an advance from traditional manual systems like the abacus and the slide rule. In 1936–7, Alan Turing conceived the idea of a modern computer. During World War II, a huge computer called Colossus was used at Bletchley Park to decipher German military codes. At first, a computer was a massive entity that was used in limited ways in industrial or military establishments.

In the 1950s, the population did not own personal computers, laptops, or mobile phones. Television was available, but in black and white transmission only. Nevertheless, computers – large bulky machines – were increasingly exerting an influence on day-to-day life, with fears about loss of jobs due to computerisation. A popular US comedy film made in 1957, *Desk Set*, portrayed the relationship between a female head of a television network's research department and a male computer consultant who was appointed to computerise her department and presumably cause her and her colleagues to be made redundant. Although the film had a happy ending, fear of redundancy due to advances in technology has not disappeared, but increased.

Personal computers became available from the mid-1970s and became widely used from the 1980s. In 1988, Michael S. Mahoney analysed the history of computing in the USA, stating that the computer had played a central role in turning the US into an information society, encouraging many different views of how information can be communicated. However, he argued that the history of computing was not being given sufficient attention within the overall history of technology, and that discussions of computing were dominated by uncritical, episodic, polemical accounts.

Mobile phones were introduced in the mid-1980s and became ubiquitous, now serving as mini computers as well as telephones. Computers have brought us a more technically advanced means of communication. In the twenty-first century, access to a personal computer gives individuals the capacity to access a range of information, and send and receive text and email messages. Personal computers connect to the *internet* – a global computer information and communication network that provides vast information and communication facilities. Communication opportunities offered by social media such as Facebook, Twitter, Instagram, Snapchat, YouTube, Reddit, Tumblr, Pinterest, Vine, Google and other internet-based organisations are popular, providing individuals with 'social networks' to share personal information linked via the internet.

Some of this communication has beneficial outcomes. Families separated by miles can keep in touch easily, and quickly convey important messages. Many people have found online shopping convenient and time-saving, without the expense of car parking, bus or train fares. Driverless cars are being developed, and robots that can perform household tasks. Town centres are diminished by the popularity of online shopping, with many well-known chain stores closing, leading to what some people fear will be the death of the high street. Email and mobile phone apps are accessed for news and information, and sales of newspapers and magazines have declined.

Yet the ways in which some technologies are being used can cause harm. E-mail or text messages written in haste and quickly posted online can be threatening to others, or reveal more than the sender really wished to convey. A frequent comment is that people nowadays spend most of their time looking at computers, both at work and at home – and walk around looking at their mobile phones rather than noticing the people around them. One might ask whether the development of this technology opens up the world or narrows it down. We can have 'friends' online whom we never meet in person. The question is asked: do these developments signal the end of communities as we know them?

Artificial intelligence (AI)

Artificial intelligence (AI) is a computer application that is having a marked effect on human society. AI – sometimes called *machine intelligence* or *computational intelligence* demonstrated by machines – consists of *intelligent agents,* devices that note their environments and take actions to achieve their goals (Poole et al., 1998). From the 1950s, the US Department of Defence funded ongoing AI research, and by the 1980s, both research and product developments had become worldwide. At the turn of the twenty-first century, as computers increased their capabilities, AI developed by firms like Google, Apple, and Microsoft influenced the way we use statistics, and study economics and mathematics. AI uses algorithms – instructional sets of data that are implemented by computers (Russell and Norvig, 1994). AI applications include development of driverless vehicles and health care technology. Artificial Intelligence (AI) is now increasingly used to generate technical 'evidence' for making professional decisions. An issue to ponder is whether communication in which artificial intelligence plays a part is beneficial or harmful to humankind. AI seems to promise more factual, accurate and speedier methods to enhance professional judgement. Yet practitioners should be aware of ethical concerns about how society uses the technology of artificial intelligence.

Ethical concerns

Key issues about the potential bias of AI have been raised by numerous scientists and writers. In 1976, Joseph Weizenbaum, a German-American computer scientist, expressed concern about computers removing human compassion from decision-making. In 1992, the American scientist Hubert Dreyfus was critical of AI, stating that one of the advantages of human expertise is that it makes use of unconscious instincts and intuition rather than being limited to precise knowledge. He argued that using AI could lead to unpredicted and unintended consequences that might cause harm. Nick Bostrom (2014), a scientist at Oxford University, also has written widely about possible negative implications of using AI.

Ric Hood, a social work academic (2018, p. 191), discussed how problem-solving increasingly uses AI to gather and process large-scale data to produce an algorithm – a set of rules or procedures for solving a problem or making a decision. The ethical danger lies in assuming that all problems are technical and that technical skill can solve all problems. Will algorithms replace professional judgement? Hari (2017) calls this 'data-ism'. It can be argued that when humans put 'garbage in', they will get 'garbage out' (Wastell and White, 2010).

Max Tegmark (2018), president of the Future of Life Institute (founded to research the impact and attendant risks of AI on economics, laws, and ethics), advocates research into AI safety. Tegmark is concerned about what might happen if a driverless car should crash, or a pacemaker fail, or an airplane crash due to technological failures. Warning of the dangers of an arms race of autonomous weapons, he nevertheless recognises the power of AI to promote good while pointing out its potential for causing harm. AI does not possess human emotions like love or fear, and it could potentially be programmed to carry out harmful actions. AI could develop destructive methods for achieving a 'good' goal. We have no means of predicting how it will behave. The Family Life Institute recommends that humans need to manage AI with wisdom, and support AI safety research.

Unintentional bias

Several commentators have warned about the problems of unintentional bias resulting when artificial intelligence is used to compile databases. In 2018, Kenan Malik, writing in the *Guardian*, portrayed the pitfalls of relying on AI, citing Amazon's abandonment of a new AI system intended to automate its recruitment processes. It was discovered that the AI system was awarding five stars to male applicants and only one star to women applicants. This AI system had been set up using previous data about recruitment decisions over the previous ten years, and it was biased in favour of male applicants because of the misogynistic nature of previous 'good' recruitment decisions. Malik argues that the ethical issue does not lie with AI itself, but with the social contexts and flawed human judgements that are used for AI programming. He concludes that artificial intelligence may generate speedy results, but humans are better at using ethical standards to challenge unintended injustices.

Gershgorn (2018) drew attention to a case where the president of the National Association for the Advancement of Coloured People (NAACP) Legal Defence Fund argued that authorities should address the bias of police and criminal justice systems which automated systems fail to recognise. Facial recognition systems are proven to be less accurate when used on individuals with darker skin; and the New York City police gang database is over-populated with ethnic minorities. Virginia Eubanks (2018) exposed human bias in the way calls for help in foster care were reported and referred for full investigations. Many more black and bi-racial families are referred for full investigations than white families. Structural bias was evident because of the flawed decisions on which the database was compiled.

Vikram Dodd, Police and Crime Correspondent for the *Guardian*, commented in 2018 that a review for the mayor of London found that too many black people are listed on a database that predicts the likelihood of people offending or becoming a victim. The database contains the details of thousands of people whom the Metropolitan Police claimed were at risk of committing gang violence or becoming victims. The Met has been given a year to reform the matrix. The review found that 38 per cent of people listed were assessed as posing no risk of committing violence. Amnesty International criticised the matrix for stigmatising black young people and ignoring human rights. The review stated that the possibility of conscious or unconscious bias against young black males in London had to be acknowledged.

Uncritical acceptance of computing and artificial intelligence

Other commentaries provide examples of computing and artificial intelligence's interference in democratic processes, or its uncritical acceptance by government and business. Naughton (2018), writing in the *Observer*, drew attention to Russian interference in democratic processes, citing the US Senate Select Committee on Intelligence's revelation that revealed that Russia's Internet Research Agency used 'disinformation techniques' to stir up distrust and confusion in social media users to encourage rightwing voters to become confrontational and provide 'fake news'. Naughton also criticised the tendency of the British government and British public to overlook the pitfalls of accepting AI without any critical evaluation, citing the Reuters Institute for the Study of Journalism's investigation of UK media coverage of AI, which found that coverage is non-critical, dominated by the computer industry, and assumes that AI provides practical solutions to human problems without considering the possible negative implications of AI.

Varadkar and Steiglitz: will computing and AI lead to more inequality?

Politicians and economists have expressed fears that the growth of computing and artificial intelligence will lead to loss of jobs and more inequality. Leo Varadkar, the Taoiseach of Ireland, warned that artificial intelligence and robots could pose risks to people's employment (Ryan, 2018), because most jobs are 'vulnerable to digitalisation or automatisation' and the important task is to think ahead. He said that about 16 per cent of men in Ireland drive for a living, and if that is automated, jobs will be lost. He suggested that the government should try to 'do something different in workforce training, supporting and incentivising employers to make sure their staff are upskilled'.

Joseph Steiglitz, Nobel Laureate and former Chief Economist at the World Bank, discussed his concerns about how AI will affect our lives (Sample, 2018). Concerned about the future of employment, he argues that although we may end up with a richer society and shorter working hours, the pitfalls of AI include routine exploitation of people's lives, a more divided society, and threats to democracy. He advises that AI and robotisation must be well-managed. Citing the Bank of England's Chief Economist, Andy Haldane, who warned that 'large swathes' of the workforce may face unemployment because of automation caused by AI, Steiglitz notes that Haldane did not say much about the possibility of new job creation. Jobs that are likely to be lost are low skilled: drivers, cashiers, call centre workers – but Steiglitz asserts there is a demand for unskilled workers in education, health and social care, however the wages are low.

Steiglitz recommends a focus on public policy issues – for example, that technological firms are able to extract and analyse data from people searching and messaging their friends online, and that sets of data can be combined so retailers can track 'customers' through their mobile phones, thus raising questions about breaches of privacy. Steiglitz is against actions that exploit people. He states that governments and technology firms have not done enough to prevent these abuses. He claims that the USA has been willing to leave technological firms to develop and enforce rules of behaviour, rather than get involved in complex technical issues. However, Stieglitz thinks that this policy is changing because of growing public awareness of how firms can use data to target customers. Stieglitz proposes setting up public regulatory structures that include specific requirements about the kinds of data technological firms can store, establishing transparency about what these firms do with the data, curbing monopoly powers and redistributing the wealth acquired by the leading AI firms. He fears that a great deal of wealth in the hands of few people leads to an unequal society. He wants more taxes, but also more labour bargaining power, more intellectual property rights, stringent competition laws, more corporate governance and changes to financial systems. If these measures are put in place, Stieglitz claims that AI could create a more prosperous, more equal society with shorter working hours, but first he recommends more public debate and decisions about how we use AI.

Nemitz: how can AI be designed to strengthen constitutional democracy?

Paul Nemitz, Principal Advisor, Directorate General for Justice and Consumers at the European Commission Brussels Area, Belgium, suggests that AI should maintain and strengthen constitutional democracy (2018). In his view, AI's capabilities – its 'big data' and 'devices of 'the Internet of all things' – increasingly govern our society's education, health, science, business, law, security, defence, politics and decision making. He identifies three characteristics: *human rights, democracy*, and the *rule of law* as core elements of democratic government constitutions, and then argues that AI must be designed to strengthen these three characteristics. He advocates setting up a new culture of technology and business development to ensure that AI capabilities will respect constitutional principles and law.

Nemitz discusses the activities of organisations which he calls the 'Frightful Five': Google, Facebook, Microsoft, Apple, and Amazon. He characterises them as profitable organisations which have access to lawmakers and wield influence over politics, civil society, science, journalism and business, yet their output is largely unregulated. He wants a debate to take place about AI, ethics and the law, because he thinks the technological firms have gained too much power over human life, putting technology above democracy in ways that contradict principles of individual freedom. He points out that internet use includes activities like mass surveillance, recruitment to terrorism, and incitement to racial hate and violence.

Nemitz considers the European Union's General Data Protection Regulation (GDPR, discussed in Chapter 8) as the first piece of legislation for AI that will explore civil responsibility levels, personal data processing, and technology impacts on human lives. He recommends establishing three levels of impact assessments for the law governing technology:

1   A parliamentary technology impact assessment at the level of policy making and legislation (to take place ideally before the deployment of high-risk technologies) in order to discover whether a technology touches on essential interests and then consider what legislation should be enacted to guarantee the public interest for that particular context.
2   An impact assessment at the level of the developers and users of this technology. These impact assessments at developer and user level would underpin public knowledge and understanding of AI, that currently lacks transparency about AI's capabilities and impacts. Impact assessments would help corporate leaders and engineers acknowledge their use of power, and help promote a technological culture of democratic responsibility, the rule of law and fundamental human rights. When AI is used to exercise public power or for public use, the impact assessment would have to be publicly available.
3   Individuals who are concerned about how AI is used should have a legal right to an explanation of AI's functions, use of logic, and how AI affects individual interests.

Nemitz believes AI needs strong rules, and self-regulatory ethics alone will not resolve the problems. AI developers should be required to consider how its products might affect democracy, fundamental human rights, and the rule of law. Otherwise, Nemitz argues, the public will have a diminishing trust in technology and AI, and there are risks to our democratic freedoms.

Impact on the public, including clients, service users, and patients

As a society, we need to ask ourselves: what do we want to use technology, computers, AI and the media for? Who controls the data that is generated? To whom does the data belong? Professional practitioners use computers in their day-to-day work. They draw on stored confidential data on their clients, patients, and users of services, and they generate more and more confidential data. Preserving confidentiality and putting safeguards in place that prevent indiscriminate use of data are pressing needs.

Availability of automated information technology (IT) systems makes communication easier for many, including banking systems that are available online, ordering groceries online, or purchasing event tickets online. Increasingly, members of the public are expected to communicate via information technology, but not all individuals want or are able to use IT as their main method of communication.

- Not all individuals have access to IT.
- They may not own a device with an internet connection because of the expense, poor internet signal, or their own lack of confidence and knowledge about how to use the technology.
- They may not wish to use the internet for banking, for example, because they worry about possible breaches of security.
- Others depend on public libraries to access the internet, but cutbacks in public expenditure have reduced library opening hours and have disadvantaged these people.

Impersonal systems

IT systems can be efficient and cost effective, but they are impersonal. One criticism of IT systems is that they lack humanity. The professional practitioner needs to keep this thought in mind when communicating with a client. Sometimes people want to hear a human voice rather than an automated system that asks them to press different digits or key in a numerical code. Technology also has its flaws. For example, voice recognition systems may not be able to recognise regional or strong accents. Another criticism of IT systems is that some people and organisations use IT technology to take advantage of individuals. Personal information can be 'hacked' to steal personal details, money, and threaten individuals. 'Fake news' destroys faith in the media and leads to questions about trust and betrayal.

Practitioners' use of information technology

Professional practitioners use information technology as a communication tool, to contact their clients and provide information and reminders of appointments. For example, the text messages that the NHS uses to remind patients of their next appointments are popular and helpful, particularly for people living alone. An isolated individual will feel less alone when they receive these reminder texts. A more complex use of technology is the development of therapy delivered by mobile phone apps. The client relationship is not with a person but with a robot.

Practice Example 10.1: How a 'chatbot' can assist with counselling

An article in Therapy Today (Brown, 2018) describes how artificial intelligence technology has created 'Woebot' – a USA-designed animated therapy 'chatbot' available as an app on mobile phones. Woebot offers a type of cognitive behavioural therapy for depression and anxiety, but is careful to remind clients that it is a robot, not a human. Brown asserts that some people are more apt to open up about their problems when they communicate with a robot, because they are not afraid of being criticised. Woebot's developers claim to be able to communicate with hard-to-reach groups that cannot be helped by other means – e.g. Syrian refugees in Lebanon. Woebot can apparently also offer compassion-focussed, emotion-focussed, interpersonal psychotherapy, mindfulness, and psychodynamic therapy, and can identify older adults' problems, including isolation, loneliness, grief, depression and anxiety. Woebot, it is claimed, may also be used for suicide prevention for men, because it is thought that men find it easier to confide in a machine. Brown comments that the Woebot programme is self-funded by an American artificial intelligence firm as a 'conscious capitalism' model. She envisions Woebot being used as an 'intelligent hold' whilst waiting to speak with a professional practitioner. Brown claims that chatbots add value as an adjunct to therapy sessions. The article gives a public relations boost to the AI bot, but Brown does mention that the AI 'brain' may adopt the biases of the humans it learns from – e.g. racism, homophobia, sexism – and can result in prejudicial decision making. Brown mentions the benefits of AI rather more than concerns about data protection and breaches of privacy. She suggests that clinicians, insurance companies and AI developers need to work closely together to develop and follow ethical guidelines, but does not mention the need for legal regulation. I query whether systems of ethics can provide sufficient safeguards for human rights without being accompanied by a legal system that promotes justice.

Ethical and legal issues for practitioners

Professional practitioners are faced with ongoing requirements to keep their IT skills up to date as part of their day-to-day work. These are the technical demands which must be met, but practitioners also need to be aware of the possible ethical and legal pitfalls of communicating via IT. Professional bodies vary in the amount of guidance they offer.

- The National Association of Social Workers in the USA published a commentary (Nielson, 2019) on communicating with purpose. The commentary explores different uses of emails, including 'revenge email', and advises against writing and sending an email when feeling emotionally upset. Neilson suggests using pen and paper instead, and then a shredder, pointing out that harsh words can have detrimental effects. The impact of hastily sent overly emotional emails can damage a practitioner's credibility or trustworthiness. Similarly, Neilson advises caution when using social media, because social media communicates instantly and once sent, the message is irrevocable. Self-awareness and social awareness should guide the words a practitioner chooses for email and social media messages.
- The British Association of Counselling and Psychotherapy (BACP, 2018) conducted a member survey in 2018 about how members used IT in their professional work, and found that 77 per cent of the respondents used digital technology for administrative and therapeutic purposes – email, texts, video conferencing, Facetime, YouTube,

Zoom and other technologies. Most of the respondents stated that they had received no training for using the technology in their professional practice.

- The British Association of Social Workers (BASW) published a policy on the use of social media (2018) to clarify BASW's views of social workers' and social work students' professional responsibilities for using social media. BASW spells out the opportunities, challenges, and risks that social media pose, especially for vulnerable people. BASW encourages use of social media for positive purposes of networking, communication, and inclusive practice, but warns that ethical dilemmas must be recognised. Social workers should be knowledgeable of technological developments and understand their impact and uses. The changes in how we communicate impacts on how practitioners collect and use information about and by individuals, and on how trust, privacy and confidentiality can be maintained in relationships with users of services. BASW wants to promote 'e-professionalism' – the ability to use and understand social media and how to manage 'the online persona of an individual based on the meaning of their online postings and interactions, including blogs, images, videos, tweets, and more'. The policy reminds social workers and students that when they are online they represent their profession and employer, and should be aware of how their communications will be received. BASW advocates professionally appropriate use of technology, including ensuring that personal communications and professional communications are kept separate, and responsible use that preserves confidentiality and privacy.
- The Health and Care Professions Council (HCPC, 2018) published guidance for its registrants and students on communicating via social media which contains 'top tips'. These tips include: thinking before posting messages, thinking about how information is shared, keeping to professional boundaries, maintaining confidentiality, not posting inappropriate material, adhering to one's employer's social media policy, and seeking advice for professional quandaries about social media communication. The guidance relates its advice to the HCPC Standards of Conduct, Performance and Ethics, advising communication to be appropriate, honest and trustworthy, based on professional judgement, respecting confidentiality, and keeping relationships with service users and carers professional.

Summarising the discussion

The future will bring expansions of technology, with increased use of social media and new applications of artificial intelligence. Instead of accepting these new developments uncritically, professional practitioners are urged to think carefully about the power implications and ethical concerns triggered by the ways we use technology and social media. Professional bodies will need to continue their development of appropriate ethical guidelines. Professional practitioners could begin by asking wider questions about how the new technology that makes communication so easy can be compatible with our democratic systems, and not potentially harm members of the public.

References

Bostrom, Nick (2014) *Superintelligence: Paths, Dangers, Strategies*. Oxford University Press: Oxford.

British Association of Counselling and Psychotherapy (BACP) (2018) *Digital technology: Love it or hate it – it's here to stay*. Accessed 15 December 2018, https://www.bacp.co.uk/events-and-re sources/ethics-and-standards/good-practice-in-action/digital-technology-survey/

British Association of Social Workers (BASW) (2018) *BASW Social Media Policy*. Accessed 5 December 2018, https://www.basw.co.uk/resources/basws-social-media-policy

Brown, Sally (2018) 'Meet the chatbots doing your job', *Therapy Today*June. Volume 29, Issue 5, pp. 8–11.

Copeland, Jack (2006) *Colossus: The Secrets of Bletchley Park's Codebreaking Computers*. Oxford University Press: Oxford.

Dodd, Vikram (2018) 'Met's gangs matrix may discriminate against black Londoners', *The Guardian*, Saturday, 22 December.

Dreyfus, Hubert L. (1992) *What Computers Still Can't Do. A Critique of Artificial Reason*. MIT Press: Cambridge MA.

Eubanks, Virginia (2018) *Automating Inequality*. St Martin's Press: New York.

Future of Life Institute (2018) *Benefits and risks of Artificial Intelligence*. *25/12/2018*. Accessed 25 January 2019, https://futureoflife.org/banckground/benefits-risks-of-artificial-intelligence

Gershgorn, Dave (2018) Algorithms can't fix societal problems and often amplify them, 17 Oct 2018. Accessed 6 December 2018, https://qz.com/1427159/algorithms-cant-fix-societal-problems-and-often-amplify-them/

Goodwin, Doris Kearns (2005) *Team of Rivals: The Political Genius of Abraham Lincoln*. Simon and Schuster: New York.

Hari, Johann (2018) *Lost Connections. Uncovering the real causes of depression – and the unexpected solutions*. Bloomsbury Publishing: London.

Health and Care Professions Council (2018) *Guidance of the use of social media*. Accessed 2 December 2018, https://www.hcpc-uk.rog/registration/meeting-our-stabdards/guidance-on-use-of-social-media/

Hood, Rick (2018) *Complexity in Social Work*. Sage: London.

Mahoney, Michael S. (1988) *The History of Computing in the History of Technology*. Program in History of Science. Annals of the History of Computing 10: Princeton University: Princeton, NJ, pp. 113–125.

Malik, Kenan. (2018) 'What's wrong with AI? Try asking a human being'. *The Guardian*. Accessed 14 October 2018, https://www.theguardian.com/commentisfree/2018/oct/14/what-is-wrong-with-ai-try-asking-a-human-being

Naughton, John (2018) 'It's official: social media is an existential threat to our democracy'. *The Observer*, 23 December.

Naughton, John (2019) 'Don't believe the hype: how the media are unwittingly selling us an AI fantasy' *The Observer*, 13 January.

Neilson, David (2019) *Communicate with purpose*. SmartBrief, National Association of Social Workers. Accessed 20 January 2019, https://www.smartbrief.com/original/2019/01/ communicate-purpose?utm_source=brief nasw@smartbrief.com.

Nemitz, Paul (2018) 'Constitutional democracy and technology in the age of artificial intelligence'. *Royal Society. Phil. Trans. R. Soc*. A376: 2018089. Accessed 29 January 2019, http://dx.doi.org/10.1098/rsta.2018.0089

Poole, D., Mackworth, A. and Goebel, R. (1998) Computational Intelligence. *A Logical Approach*. Oxford University Press: New York.

Russell, Stuart J. and Norvig, Peter (1994*) Artificial Intelligence a Modern Approach*Pearson: New York.

Ryan, Orla (2018) 'Varadkar warns that robots and artificial intelligence pose risk to people's jobs' *Thejournal.ie*. 30 December. https://JRNL.IE/4417634.

Sample, Ian (2018) 'Joseph Steiglitz on Artificial Intelligence: we're going towards a more divided society' *The Guardian*, 8 September. Accessed 25 December 2018, https://www.theguardian.com/technology/2018/sep/08/joseph…cial-intelligence-were-going-towards-a-more-divided-society

Tegmark, Max (2018) *Life 3.0: Being Human in the Age of Artificial Intelligence*. Vintage Books/ Penguin Random House: New York.

Vidal, Gore (1984) *Lincoln*. Random House: New York.

Turing, A. M. (1937) On Computable Numbers, with an Application to the Entscheidungsproblem. *Proceedings of the London Mathematical Society*, Volume 2, Issue 42(1): 230–265. Oxford Journals.

Wastell, D. and White, S. (2010) Technology as Magic: Fetish and folly in the IT-enabled reform of children's services. In Ayre, P. and Preston-Shoot, M. (eds), *Children's Services at the Crossroads: A Critical Evaluation of Contemporary Policy for Practice*. Russell House Publishing: Lyme Regis.

Weizenbaum, Joseph (1976) *Computer Power and Human Reason: From Judgment to Calculation*. W. H. Freeman: San Francisco.

Communicating in different practice situations: diabetes, addictions, and obesity

Choosing and combining different approaches

Question: How do you choose and combine communication approaches for different practice situations?

For every chosen approach, others have to be discarded. As a practitioner, you must make an individual decision about which approach or approaches you will use.

Question: Think of a particular client/patient/user of services. Which theories and methods will you choose and combine for your practice with this individual?

In a particular moment, only you can decide. Your understanding of the person's individual personality and circumstances will influence your decision. Your degree of success in balancing your 'head' (reasoning and logic) and your 'heart' (emotions) when perceiving a situation will influence your professional judgement. You will also choose on the basis of the latest published research and accounts of practice. Reflecting on your practice experiences, and learning from these experiences, will help shape your own individual 'voice' for communication and interviewing, and enable you to develop a helpful 'internal supervisor'.

Making decisions

When you find yourself in a new and challenging situation, where you have to decide what to do to resolve a situation, a formulaic procedure is unlikely to give sufficient help to decide what to do.

Practice Example 11.1 *A professional practitioner who worked for a small charity received a late evening phone call from some university students asking for help with a young woman (unknown to them), whom they found wandering around in a seemingly disoriented state but who refused to talk. They thought she might be a student and asked the counsellor to try to find out her name and address. The counsellor first met with the students and then spoke to the young woman privately. The young woman remained silent and resisted giving any response. The counsellor spent the next 45* minutes addressing a low-key monologue to the young woman, attempting to allay her fears and gain her trust. Finally the young woman began to speak, told the counsellor she was a student, gave her name and address, and agreed to be taken home. Persistence, gentleness, and the attempt to build trust helped to resolve the situation. The reasons for the young woman's initially disoriented behaviour and refusal to speak were not revealed at that point, but she showed no signs of being intoxicated, drugged, physically ill or irrational. An appointment at the university medical centre and counselling service was made for the next day.

The counsellor who helped the young woman was clinically experienced but had never engaged with a completely silent client. Although the counsellor was not certain how to offer help, he communicated his trust and acceptance to the young woman, drawing on a person-centred approach, but at the same time checking for signs of crisis.

Overcoming possible blockages in communication

Shulman (2008), a social work academic, researched practice skills as a focus for practitioner learning. He discussed possible blockages in communication and how these could be overcome. The practice skills include

- *Reaching inside of silences:* If an individual is unusually silent when you meet with them, try to find out why by asking them in an empathetic manner.
- *Supporting the individual who wants to share sensitive, difficult topics:* Help the individual to discuss topics that are not easy for them to reveal.
- *Understanding the individual's feelings:* Demonstrate your understanding when the individual shares their feelings.
- *Dealing with the theme of authority:* When the individual becomes upset about something you did or said, support the individual to share their feelings without judging or criticising them.
- *Checking for artificial consensus:* When an individual agrees with one of your suggestions too quickly, gently ask them if they really meant what they said.

Communicating in particular situations

Practitioners' responses to clients' specific health problems (including diabetes, addictions, and obesity) illustrate how they choose and combine different communication skills, and increasingly, work in partnership with a range of professions and self-help groups. A brief discussion of each heath issue conveys the essential role of sensitive communication.

Communicating with individuals who have diabetes

Diabetes is a chronic disease with no cure, but in many instances can be managed successfully through diet, exercise, and regular insulin. Symptoms include excessive thirst, fatigue, frequent urination, weight loss, genital itching and thrush, slow healing of cuts or wounds, and blurred vision (NHS Choices, 2015). Type 1 and Type 2 are two common types of diabetes. About 10 per cent of diabetics have Type 1 diabetes, and 90 per cent have Type 2. The incidence of diabetes, particularly Type 2, is increasing in the UK.

Type 2 diabetes can be controlled through diet, exercise, monitoring blood sugar levels, and good foot care. Sometimes insulin needs to be taken daily. Type 1 diabetes patients need daily insulin injections, and must observe the required health measures. Failure to observe these health requirements may result in serious health problems, including heart disease, stroke, circulation problems, gangrene, amputation, kidney failure, and blindness.

The possibility that these health problems might occur can be frightening and may trigger anxiety and fear. The need to check blood sugar daily and maintain a disciplined life style imposes what seems to be a lifelong sentence on an individual, a sentence which many would like to escape. Young people who are diagnosed with Type 1 diabetes may struggle to comply with the necessary regime of self-care because this seems to signify the end of freedom and independence. Some people are able to adopt a self-disciplined approach to managing their disease, and feel relatively little anxiety in doing so. Others perceive diabetes as completely altering their lives so that they will never be able to escape the feelings of anxiety and impending doom that the disease seems to trigger. Diabetes can result in feelings of loss (Stroebe and Schut, 1999, 2001; Kubler-Ross, 1969) that are as profound as the feelings of loss that follow a loved one's death. Each individual needs to find a personal meaning (Frankl, 2011, 1969) for their experience of diabetes, and find sufficient courage to maintain the required health regime.

> Practice Example 11.2 An older woman who was diagnosed with Type 2 diabetes adhered to the required medical regime, followed a strict diet, and monitored her blood sugar daily. Despite keeping her diabetes under control, she regarded the disease as a lifelong sentence that took away all her enjoyment of life. She could no longer eat the food she wanted, and constantly worried about herself. She felt she was in a psychological prison, and she became depressed.

The next example shows a different reaction:

> Practice example 11.3 A man in his sixties was diagnosed with Type 2 diabetes, and also a heart condition. He had a heart valve replacement some years ago but doctors are unwilling to operate again because of his diabetes. He is aware that his life span is probably shortened by his heart condition and his diabetes. He takes a philosophic view of his health, consults his doctor regularly, finds out all he can about his health condition, and enjoys life with his family.

The third practice example portrays a young man who initially struggled with his diagnosis.

> Practice example 11.4 A young man in his early twenties, who was a Type 1 diabetic, kept forgetting to take his insulin and maintain his diet. He was frequently in and out of hospital in health crisis situations, until the NHS provided a text message service that reminds diabetics to check their blood sugar and take their insulin. The young man found this messaging service helpful for managing his disease. Subsequently he volunteered to communicate the benefits of the text service to a wider audience. He was commended and praised for his voluntary work.

These three practice examples illustrate different individual reactions to diabetes, and the importance of providing appropriate professional communication to support each person. When communicating with a diabetic person, it is important to gain an individual's trust and to be non-judgemental in your response.

The woman who felt she was in a psychological prison benefited from an understanding listening ear; the man in his sixties appreciated receiving comprehensive information about his health condition, and the young man liked receiving text messages that reminded him to check his blood sugar and take his medication. All three benefited from distinctive practice approaches that combined elements of Rogers' person-centred theory (1961) with strategies that reduced stress and anxiety, built confidence, and enabled them to explore their feelings of loss, fear, and anger. These combined approaches helped individuals with diabetes to manage the symptoms of their disease, and to feel more optimistic.

Communicating with individuals with addictions

Two broad categories of addictions are *substance addictions* (alcohol or drugs, tobacco) and *behavioural/process addictions* (compulsive gambling, sexual behaviours, eating disorders including anorexia, bulimia, and over-eating, cell phone use, internet and computer use, tanning, and over-exercise, and compulsive spending). *Process addictions* are compulsive behaviours that fall outside accepted living patterns and cause difficulties for the addicted individual's family, social relationships, employment, and finances.

Identifying 'addictive personality' characteristics can help to explain why some individuals develop addictions. The hope is that if ways and means of preventing and curing the addictions can be found, practitioners could predict who is more likely to become addicted. The concept of the 'addictive personality' (Lang, 1983) suggests that:

- An addictive personality has a set of personality traits that result in becoming predisposed to developing addictions.
- The 'trigger' causes include: biological factors (inherited, genetic); psychological factors (emotional); and environmental factors (upbringing, social circumstances).
- Indications of an addictive personality may include spending excessive time engaging in certain behaviours, acting compulsively or impulsively, the person believing that they do not fit into society, sensitivity to emotional stress; difficulty in handling frustrations; low self-esteem; mood swings, depression, insecurity about relationships; and seeking approval.

An ongoing debate continues about whether an 'addictive personality' really exists, and whether this concept labels individuals inaccurately, who then may become discouraged and begin to believe that nothing can help them to change. It is helpful to note that the use of hypnotherapy can assist practice with addictions (Heap, 2012)

Tobacco addiction

Smoking tobacco is a widespread social habit that leads to preventable deaths (about 90,000 per year in the UK). Generally regarded as an addiction, most people find it difficult to give up smoking. Smoking causes debilitating fatal diseases, such as lung cancer, coronary obstructive pulmonary disease (COPD), and heart disease. People may want to give up smoking, but much depends on their strength of motivation and receiving professional communication that supports their motivation. Obstacles to success include subconscious factors, physical addiction to the nicotine in tobacco, and emotional attachment to smoking. Hadley and Staudacher (1989, pp. 71–81) identify motivations to smoke: nurturing the self, relieving stress, ameliorating awkward social situations, and controlling weight. Heap and Alexander (2012) advise that the pleasurability of smoking diminishes motivations to quit. They suggest total abstinence as the helping goal.

> *Question:* How would you communicate with an individual who wants to give up smoking?

You can offer the individual up-to-date facts and figures on smoking, learn about their smoking history, smoking timetable, reasons for wanting to quit, family and friends' support or possible sabotage, and how the individual feels about giving up. Then you could encourage the individual to share the positive benefits of giving up (including their personal reasons). The aim is to build their motivation to become a non-smoker.

The next steps are to identify when, where, and why a person smokes, set up a smoke-free plan, and then attempt to 're-programme' the person's motivation to quit. Re-programming includes building confidence that they can reach the goal of quitting smoking, helping them to perceive smoking as unappealing and themselves as healthy, energetic non-smokers, and incorporating these new behaviour patterns into their daily routines.

An initial meeting should try to build a positive client relationship. Communication strategies will seek to establish a trusting relationship by offering acceptance, a non-judgemental attitude, and unconditional positive regard (Rogers, 1951). The practitioner will explain the kind of support than can be offered, its purpose, and how this support might help overcome the addiction, but must be honest about the scope and limitations of this strategy. The practitioner also should explore whether the client has other addictions like alcohol or substance misuse.

Gambling addictions

Television advertising in the UK communicates a positive view of gambling (sweepstakes, the lottery, etc.). Gamblers are portrayed in television advertisements as happy, successful, attractive, prosperous, and young. Gambling is represented as fun – a pleasurable activity. This kind of advertising can exert a harmful influence on vulnerable individuals, who risk being enticed into the world of gambling by misrepresentations in TV advertisements. These advertisements portray gambling as a glamorous activity, but, in actuality, motivating people to gamble is an activity that can prey on emotionally needy people.

Lesieur and Custer (1984) suggested that pathological gambling is a treatable illness, thus rejecting the Freudian theory (1986) that people gamble compulsively as a substitute for sex. They argue that gambling addiction has less to do with money than with the fear of dying and a need to 'stay alive' through gambling activity, and to escape psychological pain.

Blaszczynski and Nower (2002) developed a pathway model of problems and pathological gambling. This model organises gambling addicts' characteristics into three pathways, each with suggested helping strategies. Although its analytical approach encourages practitioners to think through possible choices, the model seems to discount the possibility of success with certain individuals.

- Pathway 1 (behaviourally conditioned problem gamblers) considers, inter alia, ecological factors of increased availability and accessibility to gambling, which can be treated effectively with counselling and minimal intervention programmes.
- Pathway 2 (emotionally vulnerable problem gamblers) considers the same characteristics but adds emotional vulnerability, which includes childhood disturbance; risk-taking, boredom, depression, anxiety; poor coping and problem solving, life stresses and substance misuse. These symptoms can be ameliorated by interventions based on *abstinence* (Blaszczynski, 2010, pp. 73–76) (where the addict is encouraged to give up their addictive behaviour entirely) rather than *harm reduction or controlled gambling* (Blaszczynski, 2010, pp. 73–76, 111–13).
- Pathway 3 (anti-social impulsivist problem gamblers) considers the same characteristics as Pathway 2, but adds impulsive traits, including ADHD (attention deficit hyperactivity disorder), impulsivity, and anti-social behaviour. These symptoms suggest that the individual is less motivated to seek help, and will respond poorly.

Prochaska and DiClemente's *cycle of change* (1986) acknowledges that relapses in motivation are likely. Their cycle aims to build understanding and motivation gradually. Steps along the way to overcoming addiction include *pre-contemplation of change, contemplation, preparation, action, maintenance*, and *relapse*.

Addicts may use defence mechanisms of *denial, rationalisation*, and *projection* of blame onto others (Freud, 1936) to make sense of their frequent relapses rather than 'owning' personal responsibility for their addictions. An addict may have a range of other problem issues, and these can sometimes distract the practitioner from identifying and intervening with the underlying 'trigger cause' – the addiction itself.

> Practice example 11.5 *A social worker tried to help a homeless man who was addicted to alcohol. He helped the man begin to manage his debts, find employment and housing, and encouraged him to reunite with his family. These attempts to help at first seemed promising but ultimately did not succeed. The man continued to drink, left his family, and became homeless again. The social worker had failed to confront the causal issue of the problems – the addiction itself. Non-compliance and relapse soon occurred.*

When you communicate with an addicted person, try to recognise the spark of humanity that links each person and do not force your own views on the individual. You can combine person-centred therapy (Rogers, 1951), psycho-dynamic therapy (Jacobs, 2006), and CBT strategies (Blaszczynski, 1998) to encourage an individual to think differently about their addictive behaviours and start to build emotional resilience that will help them sustain their efforts to change.

You should consider whether the addict's family members are 'co-dependents' (e.g. engaging in a dysfunctional helping relationship) and may also need support. In dysfunctional helping relationships, one person's help may support and enable the other person's underachievement and/or irresponsibility. The co-dependent person takes responsibility for the other person's predicaments, bears their negative consequences for them, accommodates their unhealthy or irresponsible behaviours, and takes care of them so that the other person does not develop the usual competences expected for people of their age or abilities. These co-dependent relationships tend to deplete the helper's physical, emotional, or financial resources and lead to resentment and strained relationships.

Trying to help gambling addicts requires more than one-to-one help from a single profession. A 'wrap-around' service should provide not only help to individuals, but also support services like an online forum, group support, a help line, debt advice, and reliable sources of information about how addicts can be helped. Helping gambling addicts requires multi-professional intervention with group and peer support. The UK National Gambling Help Line offers support for gambling addictions. An online forum is available to gambling addicts and their carers and families. Communication and interviewing skills play an essential part in building a therapeutic relationship that encourages an individual's motivation to tackle their addiction.

Communicating with obese individuals

Obesity is a chronic disease that can increase the incidence of heart disease, diabetes, and strokes. Easy availability of sugar-laden take-away meals, together with more sedentary life styles, contributes to increases in obesity. Obesity affects the well-being and self-esteem of an increasing range of people, including those from lower socio-economic levels. Reasons for overeating include psychological needs, parental influences, eating as a reward or entertainment, a way of decreasing or negating unpleasant experiences, a desire to be noticed and gain authority, addiction, fear of deprivation, as a substitute for love, or because of fear of sexuality, feeling unattractive, or worry about health (Leach, 2006).

Communicating with obese persons should demonstrate empathy and respect (Biestek, 1992, 1957) rather than blame or disapproval. Some individuals may not recognise their obesity as a problem and may reject attempts to help them reduce their weight. They cannot be compelled to do so. The practitioner may identify, in partnership with the individual, the circumstances of the obesity, including cultural, family, social and historical influences on body size and shape, ethnic values, social environments for eating and food; and psychological triggers that lead to overeating. Jointly exploring issues can create a shared understanding of the individual's experience of eating and relationship with food. This shared understanding is part of an empowering process that motivates individuals to change (Higham, 2009).

Developing different techniques helps practitioners tailor communication to individual characteristics. A practitioner's relationship with each individual and growing knowledge of the individual's motivation will guide the communication. To change self-destructive orientations towards food, practitioners will aim to motivate individuals to examine and challenge long-standing beliefs and habits.

- Motivational interviewing (MI) was developed for working with alcoholics, but can help with obesity and other conditions (Miller and Rollnick, 2002, Miller, 1983). Motivational interviewing is a pre-intervention communication strategy that builds constructive relationships between the individual and the practitioner, and then evaluates problem behaviours and resistance to change in the light of personal values and goals.
- Hadley and Staudacher (1989, p. 60) argue that people whose excessive weight results from overeating will not lose weight unless they consider the causes of their overeating. The practitioner can suggest pinpointing when, where, and why an individual overeats by asking them to complete a checklist of circumstances that prompt them to eat, including their feelings about eating and food, the places where they are likely to eat, and their reasons for eating.
- Leach (2006) suggested a transactional analysis-based approach for tackling obesity, She argued that obese individuals use psychological game-playing as a source of 'strokes' (units of recognition) and a defence against open communication. Berne (1964) adapted transactional analysis (TA) from psychoanalytic theory. The TA approach seeks to learn how individuals communicate through patterns of relationships and behaviours based on the three ego states of the child, the parent, and the adult. TA assumes that people are, in essence, 'OK' and their here-and-now rational adult self (adult ego state) can make positive choices, rather than allowing their negative internalised parent ego state, or fearful inner child ego state to invalidate these choices. The usefulness of this therapeutic approach depends on whether the practitioner is comfortable working with psychological causes and has appropriate skills.
- Hypnotherapy techniques, such as progressive relaxation (Jacobson, 1987), can be helpful.

Approaches based on psychological approaches tend to avoid in-depth alternative explanations for the rising incidence of obesity, for example, the decline in heavy physical activity in people's occupations, the increasing use of automobiles, the decrease in physical exercise, and food suppliers promoting fatty calorific food laden with sugar and carbohydrates.

Obesity is a relevant issue for practice. Practitioners' ability to consider environmental and contextual issues is an appropriate skill for working with obesity. By working in partnership with other professions, practitioners can help individuals to change their eating patterns that lead to obesity by communicating effectively with them. This can be a slow process. First comes the task of motivating the individual. When an obese individual is motivated to change, the practitioner might use informal educational processes, like the *social pedagogue* model – a relationship-based intervention that promotes well-being, learning and growth, believing in each individual's intrinsic worth (Kornbeck and Lumsden, 2008). The practitioner can communicate information about the health risks of obesity, including diet sheets, encouragement of healthy eating, medication, weight loss groups, and the benefits of exercise as well as offering person-centred acceptance. Public Health practitioners can be a helpful source of strategies for addressing the issues of obesity.

Summary

The chapter's discussion of mental illness, diabetes, addictions, and obesity illustrates the importance of using a range of communication strategies and engaging in multi-professional partnerships with other professional services. You will enhance your practice skills as you overcome blockages in communication and learn how to respond to individuals who are experiencing different life situations. As you develop your practice, you progress towards developing your own distinctive style, with appropriate approaches for communicating with and interviewing a range of people who seek help for a range of issues. Your continuing professional development activities, as well as your ongoing practice experience and reflective supervision, will help you to become and remain an effective practitioner.

References

Beresford, P. (2016) *All Our Welfare: Towards Participatory Social Policy*. Policy Press: Bristol.

Berne, Eric (1964) *Games People Play. The psychology of human relationships*. Grove Press: New York.

Biestek, F. (1992, 1957) *The Casework Relationship*. Routledge: London.

Blaszczynski, Alex (2010) *Overcoming Compulsive Gambling*. Robinson: London.

Blaszczynski, Alex, and Nower, Lia (2002) 'A pathways model of problem and pathological gambling' *Addiction*, Volume 97, pp. 487–499.

Blaszczynski, A. (1998) *Overcoming compulsive gambling: a self-help guide using cognitive behavioral techniques*. Robinson: London.

Campbell, J. and Oliver, M. (1996) *Disability politics: understanding our past, changing our future*. Routledge: London.

Frankl, V. (2011, 1969) *Man's Search for Ultimate Meaning*. Basic Books: Cambridge, MA.

Freud, A. (1936, 2018) *The Ego and the Mechanisms of Defense*. Routledge: Abingdon.

Freud, S. (1986 edition) *The Essentials of Psycho-Analysis* (selected by Anna Freud). Penguin: London.

Goffman, E. (1961) *Asylums: Essays on the Social situation of Mental Patients and Other Inmates*. Anchor Books: New York.

Hadley, J. and Staudacher, C. (1989) *Hypnosis for Change*. New Harbinger Publications: Oakland CA.

Heap, Michael (editor) (2012) *Hypnotherapy. A Handbook*. 2nd Edition. Open University Press: Maidenhead, Berkshire.

Heap, M. and Alexander, D. (2012) 'Hypnotherapy and smoking, weight loss, and alcohol and drug abuse' in M. Heap (ed.), *Hypnotherapy. A Handbook*, Open University Press, McGraw-Hill Education: Maidenhead.

Higham, P. (2009) 'Options against obesity', *Professional Social Work*, March, pp. 26–27.

Jacobs, M., (2006) *The Presenting Past: The Core of Psychodynamic Counselling and Therapy*. 3rd Edition. Open University Press: Milton Keynes.

Jacobson, E. (1987) 'Progressive Relaxation', *The American Journal of Psychology*, Volume 100, Issue 3/4, Special Centennial Issue (Autumn–Winter), pp. 522–537.

Kornbeck, J. and Lumsden, E. (2008) European skills and models. The relevance of the social pedagogue. In P. Higham, *Post-Qualifying Social Work Practice*. Sage: London, 122–132.

Kubler-Ross, E. (1969) *On Death and Dying*. Macmillan: New York.

Lang, Alan R. (1983) 'Addictive Personality. A Viable Construct?' In Levison, Peter K., Gerstein, DeanR., Maloff, DeborahR. *Commonalities in Substance Abuse and Habitual Behavior*. Lexington Books: Lanham, MD, pp. 157–236.

Leach, K. (2006) *The Overweight Patient. A Psychological Approach to Understanding and Working with Obesity*. Jessica Kingsley: London

Lesieur, H. L., and Custer, R. L. (1984) 'Pathological Gambling: Roots, Phases, and Treatment' *Gambling: Views from the Social Sciences* (July), Volume 474, pp. 146–156.

Miller, W. (1983) 'Motivational Interviewing with problem drinkers', *Behavioural Psychotherapy*, Volume 11, pp. 147–172.

Miller, W.R. and Rollnick, S. (2002) *Motivational Interviewing: Preparing People for Change*. 2nd Edition Guilford Press: New York.

Neimeyer, Robert A. (2009) *Constructivist Psychotherapy*. Routledge: London.

NHS Choices (2015) (a) *Living with Diabetes*. Accessed online 11 July 2015.

Prochaska, J.O. and DiClemente, C. C. (1986) 'Toward a comprehensive model of change' in Prochaska, J. A. *Treating Addictive Behaviours*, pp. 3–27. Springer: New York.

Rogers, C. (1951) *Client-Centered Therapy: Its Current Practice, Implications and Theory*. Constable: London.

Rogers, C. R. (1961) *On Becoming a Person*. Constable: London.

Shulman, L. (1984) *The Skills of Helping: Individuals and Groups*. 2nd Edition. F.E. Peacock: Itasca, Illinois.

Shulman, L. (2008) *The Skills of Helping: Individuals and Groups*. 6th Edition. F.E. Peacock: Itasca, Illinois.

Stroebe, M. S. and Schut, H. (1999) 'The dual process model of coping with bereavement: Rationale and description', *Death Studies*, Volume 23, pp. 197–211.

Stroebe, M. S. and Schut, H. (2001) 'Meaning making in the dual process model of coping with bereavement' in R.A. Neimeyer (ed.), *Meaning Reconstruction and the Experience of Loss*. American Psychological Association: Washington, D. C., pp. 55–73.

Chapter 12

Communicating in situations of loss

Situations of loss and mourning

Understanding how to communicate in situations of loss and mourning is a key skill for professional practitioners. Many people in our society would acknowledge that discussing death and bereavement is a task that most individuals find hard to face. It is said that loss and mourning have replaced sexuality as a taboo subject. Victorian society was acquainted with death as an everyday event, because of high infant mortality rates and short life expectancies. Increasingly, during the nineteenth and twentieth centuries, advancements in sanitation and health care led to an increase in infant survival and life expectancy. People push out of their minds the fact that we will all die some day and that death is a certainty. Human beings have developed collective amnesia about the reality of death.

Feelings of loss

Feelings of loss are triggered not just by the occurrence of a death, but by other kinds of loss, encountered through divorce, illness, ageing, unemployment, retirement, sexual abuse, death of a pet, change of school, moving house, children leaving home, and broken relationships. Of these, death is the most difficult loss to discuss openly, but all kinds of loss can be difficult for individuals to face and acknowledge.

Feelings of grief and loss occur when a loved one dies, but also when valued relationships, roles, identities and skills are lost. Religious faith can cushion the impact of losses, but fewer people in contemporary Britain profess religious beliefs. Modern medicine's success means that the population no longer experiences death as an everyday occurrence. People used to die at home. Now most people die in hospitals or nursing homes, away from society's gaze. Individuals may deny their feelings of loss, or acquaintances may avoid discussing the loss.

Practitioners should learn how to recognise feelings of loss and mourning that may underpin a person's reactions and then communicate sensitively and with discretion. Even when they do, the individual may not want to respond. Sometimes theoretical interpretations of behaviour are rejected.

> Practice example 12.1: *A mother of a ten-year-old boy reported his behavioural problems to her social worker, and asked for help. After developing trust in the social worker, she confided that her father had died suddenly in an accident when she was twelve years old, and she remembered quarrelling with him as he left for work on the day of the accident. That was the last time she saw him. After the social*

worker felt that a relationship of trust had been established, she suggested that perhaps the mother had felt anger, guilt and grief about her father's death and now those feelings perhaps were being directed towards her son.

The social worker drew on Freudian theories of transference (2018, 1936) in her response, as well as using a person-centred approach (Rogers, 1951). The mother listened to the practitioner's suggestion, but politely rejected the offer to discuss her relationship with her deceased father, preferring to focus solely on her feelings about her son's behaviour.

Theories that try to explain loss and mourning

Humphrey and Zimpfer (2008, pp. 4–9) suggest that many grief and loss theories evolved from Bowlby's attachment theory rather than developing different conceptual models – portraying grieving and loss as stages, concepts, tasks, processes and phases. Theory development began with Freud (1914), who argued that mourning involves a search for a lost attachment, and that the ego eventually must disengage from the lost person or object. Later, Lindeman's empirical research (1944) on grief reactions to the deaths caused by the Boston Coconut Grove nightclub fire identified symptoms of 'normal' grief and 'pathological' grief.

Elisabeth Kubler-Ross (1969), a psychoanalytically oriented psychiatrist, developed a secular explanation of grief and loss reactions. Conducting interviews with over 200 dying patients, she suggested five stages of grief and loss reactions: *denial, anger, bargaining, depression,* and *acceptance.* Current thinking suggests that these stages do not always occur sequentially, nor does every individual move through each stage (Stephenson, 1985).

Theoretical contributions that consider a wider range of losses include:

- Bowlby's theory of attachment behaviour (1969, 1973, 1980), which claims that attachment is instinctive, and identifies *numbing, yearning and searching, disorganisation and despair* and *reorganisation* as four phases of reactions to loss.
- Colin Murray-Parkes (1972), who drew attention to the social transitions that took place during bereavement, argued that human beings construct the world around them and create an 'assumptive world'. Murray-Parkes constructed stages of bereavement that included numbness (denial), yearning/longing, realisation, and acceptance, suggesting that these stages represent a journey on which the individual will embark in order to resolve their grief.
- Worden (2002) identified four tasks for individuals experiencing loss and bereavement: accept the reality of the loss; work through the pain of grief; adjust to a world in which the dead person is missing, and emotionally relocate the dead person and move on.
- Rando's six 'R' processes (1993) of mourning – the *avoidance* phase, when the bereaved person must *recognise* the loss and achieve understanding; the *confrontation* stage, when the bereaved person *reacts* to the separation, *recollects* and *re-experiences* the relationship with the dead person, and then *relinquishes* old attachments; and the *accommodation* phase that includes *readjusting* to a new world and *reinvesting* in life.

Until recently, the efficacy of these 'stage theories' of loss and mourning was widely accepted, but now newer existential cognitive theories of loss that critique the Kubler-Ross and other 'stage theory' approaches have become popular. These include *continuing bonds* theory (Silverman and Klass, 1996; Silverman and Nickman, 1996); the *dual process* model (DPM) (Stroebe and Schut, 1999, 2001); and *constructivism* (Neimeyer, 2001). The newer theories raise doubts about whether stage theories provide a broad enough understanding of loss. Stage theories can be problematic, because some individuals exhibit behaviour and feelings that get 'stuck' at a particular stage (for example, numbness, denial or anger).

Kubler-Ross, Bowlby, Murray-Parkes, Worden and Rando accepted Freud's psychoanalytic views, and like Freud, argued that the grieving person must 'move on' from their loss. More recent theoretical models like *continuing bonds* theory, the *dual process*, and *constructivism* disagree with Freudian concepts of 'pathological grieving' and 'moving on', and instead try to help individuals accommodate loss within their ongoing lives. These models focus on working in partnership with clients to help them accommodate the loss in their lives, rather than urging them to 'move on' after the loss.

Question: How often have you observed a completed cycle of stages of loss in one individual?

- *Continuing bonds* theories (Silverman and Klass, 1996; Silverman and Nickman, 1996) reject the idea that successful grief resolution requires disengaging from the dead person, and argue instead that individuals experience a process of adaptation and change in their relationship with the dead person, and then construct and reconstruct new connections that maintain a significant but changed relationship with the dead person (Silverman and Klass, 1996, p. 18). Successful resolution is keeping a loving memory and representation of the dead individual – a changed kind of relationship with different kinds of gratification. Bereaved individuals maintain a significant but changed relationship with the dead person.
- The *dual process* model (DPM) (Stroebe and Schut, 1999, 2001 suggests that two stress points occur after a death: *loss orientation* (grieving) and *restoration orientation* (dealing with practical issues). The dual process model asserts that grief manifests itself in two ways: preoccupation with resolving the practical issues posed by the loss of a loved one, and the emotional reactions to loss. Stroebe and Schut (1999, 2001) criticise other models for ignoring gender roles, cultural differences, and social support, and lacking empirical evidence and clarity. The model suggests two stress points occur after a death: *loss orientation* (grieving) and *restoration orientation* (dealing with practical issues). Stroebe and Schut suggest that grieving individuals process grief and move from a loss-orientated position to one of *restoration*.

Practice example 12. 2 The husband of a seventy-year-old woman had recently died after a long illness of Parkinson's disease and dementia. His widow related every detail of his memorial service arrangements, sorting out finances, and disposing of his possessions, saying how tired and stressed she felt from undertaking these activities. The counsellor listened empathetically and mentioned the Dual Process Model (*Stroebe and Schut, 1999,* 2001) as a way of affirming the normality of her emotions and fatigue. He suggested that when the widow's tasks were completed, she might like to give herself a 'treat'. He could not tell her what that treat might be, it had to be of her own choosing. At that moment, he felt that she paused, looked at him intensely and responded positively to his suggestion.

- Constructivism (Neimeyer, 2001) suggests that a key process for resolving grief is to reconstruct the meaning of one's relationship with the dead person. Neimeyer's constructivism suggests that mourners construct a statement that explains the loss and use this construction to help them recover from the loss. The process of reconstructing relationships recognises individuals' resilience – that they can recover from loss and find new meanings in life. Neimeyer (2001) criticises previous theories that emphasise 'letting go' of the relationship, arguing that reconstruction of meaning is an important grieving process. He suggests that instead of Kubler-Ross' view (1969) of loss and mourning – that the individual simply 'moves on' from the relationship – the individual reconstructs their relationship with the person who has died or who is no longer close.

Practice Example 12.3 *After her husband died, the woman remembered him as a wise, engaging supportive presence in her life: 'Oh, I do miss him, we had such wonderful conversations together.' She left out years of quarrelling and depression and mentioned only the positive aspects of their relationship.*

Victor Frankl's Logotherapy

Frankl's *logotherapy*, which emphasises a search for meaning and individual insights into loss, also provides important understanding. Neimeyer links Frankl's search for meaning to his constructivism. Frankl (1969) rejected Freudian theory and the behavioural view that humans are products of their environment (Butler-Bowdon, 2007). This approach is relevant to theories of loss and mourning.

Viktor Frankl was a Jewish Viennese psychiatrist who, after surviving two Nazi concentration camps where his wife and daughter died, developed his system of logotherapy. *Logotherapy* is a search for meaning that encourages individual insight on loss and bereavement, recognises the individual's capacity to sustain dignity in the midst of crisis, acknowledges spiritual conflicts about guilt and death, and accepts that spiritual leaders may be more effective than psychiatrists for helping individuals resolve their grief. (Frankl argued that religion is concerned with salvation, and logotherapy is concerned with mental health.)

Logotherapy promotes individual human responsibility and accepts the reality of human guilt. Frankl argued that each individual has a unique set of potential meanings to their life, and each individual must decide whether to accept or avoid those meanings. There is no ultimate 'meaning of life', but instead, individual meanings of individual lives. Frankl believed that individual life – including suffering and loss – has meaning. Although people may have difficulty understanding the meaning of their life when they experience difficult situations, it is possible to achieve eventual understanding. Frankl thought that the greatest human achievement is to face one's fate with courage, a relevant principle for working with dying and bereaved people.

> Practice example 12. 4 A social work department asked one of its social workers to visit a middle-aged woman with terminal cancer. She visited weekly and counselled the woman until the woman died, using a person-centred supportive approach (Rogers, 1951). The woman's husband and teen-aged children were caring and attentive, but the woman wanted to delve further into her feelings about her life and impending death. The social worker listened to the woman share her moments of joy when she saw trees and flowers in bloom, and other moments of recollected happiness. Her mood was contemplative rather than despairing. It occurred to the social worker that this woman was searching for meaning as part of her preparation for death.

Additional views of loss and mourning

- Bayliss (2008) argued that grief is not a disease, and suggested that when a person experiences a loss, life will never be the same again – the person will experience an erratic cycle of grief. The process of bereavement moves an individual on from the original loss, sometimes backward and forward along a line of grief. Despite hoping that life will return to normal, the individual must accept that their life will never be the same again, and that living a different life can be a good experience.
- Wallbank (1991, p. 18) used an analogy: *grief comes and goes, it flows in and out like a tide.* Just as tides flow in and out in different intensities, each individual experiences their grief differently within their particular personal and social contexts.

Communication skills for practice in situations of loss and mourning

A professional practitioner working in situations involving grief and loss is likely to adopt a person-centred approach (Rogers, 1951) to gain trust, form a therapeutic relationship, assess the individual's situation, and select an appropriate intervention to address the particular experience of loss (Reeves, 2013). A person–centred approach (Rogers, 1951) sets the individual at ease and builds confidence. Going slowly, listening carefully, and seeking to convey non-judgemental acceptance are generally effective communication strategies. The timing of when individuals choose to express their grief can be significant, with Christmas being a time when a bereaved individual can feel particularly vulnerable.

> Practice example 12.5 A consultant anaesthetist dropped into a counselling centre on Christmas Eve to offer himself as a volunteer to help teenagers. The counsellor who spoke with him wondered at first why he decided to volunteer. After talking to him, she discovered that he was a grieving father whose son had died in an incident with the police. He blamed himself for his son's death. She acknowledged his sorrow, and tried to offer an accepting response. This seemed to be what he was looking for. She felt he needed to reconstruct his belief in himself as a caring father (Neimeyer, 2001).

Reactions to bereavement and loss will vary, influenced by cultural and national identities, religious and spiritual beliefs, past relationships with the lost person or object, and the client's own emotional make-up. Some cultures express grief in an open, emotional way, whilst other cultures repress their feelings of loss. Practitioners need to accept these different expressions of sorrow. Problems in childhood attachment (Bowlby, 1969, 1973, 1980) and low self-esteem may exacerbate an individual's reactions.

> Practice example 12.6 *A teenaged boy suddenly told his counsellor that he remembered feeling nothing – being empty of emotion – at his mother's funeral as he watched her coffin being lowered into the ground. The counsellor offered acceptance, but also suggested that his numbness was in fact an expression of hidden sorrow. He did not recognise his reaction as an expression of grief, but there was an urgency and intensity in his communication about his mother.*

This young man's reaction of 'feeling nothing' seemed to illustrate the Kubler-Ross theory about the stages of loss and mourning (1969). Some grief reactions may be more complex and profound than others. Sudden bereavements resulting from natural disasters, violence, murder, the absence of a funeral ceremony, or when no human remains can be found may lead to more complex reactions that take longer to address. I prefer to call these reactions 'complex grief' rather than 'pathological grief', because I think the latter designation can appear judgemental.

The personal challenges of communicating in situations of bereavement and loss include the risk of becoming overwhelmed by people's emotions. Sustaining communication in this emotionally demanding area requires self-reflection, professional support, and ensuring that the principle of 'do no harm' is uppermost in mind. Working with loss and mourning carries the risk that an individual's traumatic experiences may result in clinical depression and thoughts of suicide. Practitioners need to exercise appropriate professional judgement for referring individuals with these presenting issues to a medical physician. The initial stage of counselling should contain a 'risk of harm' analysis to protect the individual from harm. An inexperienced practitioner may struggle to decide when to refer a client on. Professional supervision helps a practitioner to avoid potentially harmful decisions. Ethical practice requires self-reflection, learning from experience, and adherence to ethical codes. Necessary skills include knowledge of a range of theoretical models, and choosing and implementing appropriate combinations of theoretical models for each individual situation.

The following skills are important for practising in situations of loss and mourning:

- acceptance of individual experiences of loss
- awareness of your own experiences of grief and loss
- sensitivity to individual symptoms of distress
- empathetic listening skills
- responding sensitively to each individual's own unique reactions to grief and loss
- enabling a search for meaning

References

Bayliss, J. (2008) *Counselling Skills in Palliative Care*. Quay Books: Salisbury.
Bowlby, J. (1969) *Attachment and Loss, Vol. 1: Attachment*. Basic Books: New York.

Bowlby, J. (1973) *Attachment and Loss, Vol. 2: Separation: Anxiety and anger*. Basic Books: New York.

Bowlby, J. (1980) *Attachment and Loss, Vol. 3: Loss: Sadness and depression*. Basic Books: New York.

Butler-Bowdon, T. (2007) *50 Psychology Classics: Who We Are, How We Think, What We Do: Insight and Inspiration From 50 Key Books*. Nicholas Brealey: London & Boston.

Erikson, E. (1980) *Identity and the Life Cycle*. Norton: New York.

Frankl, V. (1969) *The Will to Meaning: Foundations and Applications of Logotherapy*. Meridian: London.

Freud, A. (1936, 2018) *The Ego and the Mechanisms of Defense*. Routledge: Abingdon.

Freud, S. (1914/1957) 'Mourning and melancholia', in J. Strachey (ed. and trans.), *The Standard Edition of the Complete Psychological Works of Sigmund Freud*, Volume 14. Hogarth: London.

Freud, S. (1986) *The Essentials of Psycho-analysis, selected by Anna Freud*. Penguin: London.

Jung, C. G. (1968) *The Archetypes and the Collective Unconscious*. Princeton University Press: Princeton.

Humphrey, G. and Zimpfer, David G. (2008) *Counselling for Grief and Bereavement*. Second Edition Sage: London.

Kubler-Ross, E. (1969) *On Death and Dying*. Macmillan: New York.

Lindeman, E. (1944) 'Symptomatology and management of acute grief', *American Journal of Psychiatry*, Volume 101, pp. 141–148.

Murray-Parkes, C. (1972) *Bereavement: Studies of Grief in Adult Life*. Intl. U. Press: New York.

Neimeyer, R.A. (2001) 'Introduction: Meaning reconstruction and loss', in R.A. Neimeyer (ed.), *Meaning Reconstruction and the Experience of Loss*. American Psychological Association: Washington, D.C., pp. 1–9.

Rando, T. A. (1993) *Treatment of Complicated Mourning*. Research Press: Champaign, IL.

Reeves, A. (2013) *An Introduction to Counselling and Psychotherapy (From Theory to Practice)*. Sage: London.

Rogers, C. (1951) *Client-Centered Therapy: Its Current Practice, Implications and Theory*. Constable: London.

Silverman, P. R. and Klass, D. (1996) 'Introduction: What's the problem?' in D. Klass, P.R. Silverman and S.L. Nickman (eds), *Continuing Bonds*. Taylor and Francis: Washington, D.C., pp. 4–27.

Silverman, P. R. and Nickman (1996) 'Concluding thoughts', in D. Klass, P.R. Silverman and S.L. Nickman (eds) *Continuing Bonds*. Taylor and Francis: Washington, D.C., pp. 345–355.

Stephenson, J. S. (1985) *Death, Grief and Mourning*. The Free Press: New York.

Stroebe, M. S. and Schut, H. (1999), 'The dual process model of coping with bereavement: Rationale and description', *Death Studies*, Volume 23, pp. 197–211.

Stroebe, M. S. and Schut, H. (2001) 'Meaning making in the dual process model of coping with bereavement', in R.A. Neimeyer (ed.), *Meaning Reconstruction and the Experience of Loss*. American Psychological Association: Washington, DC, pp. 55–73.

Wallbank, S. (1991) *Facing Grief: Bereavement & the Young Adult*. Lutterworth Press: Cambridge.

Worden, W. (2002) *Grief Counseling and Grief Therapy: A handbook for the mental health practitioner*. 3rd Edition). Springer: New York.

Chapter 13

Communicating in situations of domestic violence

What is domestic violence?

Refuge (a large national provider of support for women, children and men who experience domestic violence) defines domestic violence as abuse of power within an intimate or family relationship – 'systematic, patterned behaviour on the part of the abuser designed to control his or her partner' (2019, https://www.refuge.org.uk/). Domestic violence against women is a recognised occurrence, but individuals of any gender or sexuality may experience domestic violence. As well as physical and sexual abuse, domestic abuse may be non-physical and consist of psychological, verbal, emotional and financial control. The Refuge charity lists different indicators of domestic violence, giving an example of an individual changing their behaviour because they fear a partner's reactions.

The charity Women's Aid (Women's Aid, 2019, https://www.womensaid.org.uk/) defines domestic abuse similarly, but in more detail, as incidents or patterns of incidents of controlling, coercive, threatening, degrading and violent behaviour, including sexual violence, mostly by a partner or ex-partner, but also by a family member or carer. Domestic abuse can include *coercive control* (intimidation, degradation, isolation, the threat of physical or sexual violence); *psychological and/or emotional abuse; physical or sexual abuse, financial abuse, harassment and stalking*, and *online or digital abuse*. Domestic violence can include forced marriage, female genital mutilation and 'honour crimes' by family members. Alternative definitions of domestic violence include *family violence, domestic abuse, and abusive relationships.*

Browxtowe Women's Project, a charity in Nottinghamshire that offers support to women who experience domestic violence, explains domestic abuse as an incident or pattern of controlling, coercive or threatening behaviour, violence, or abuse, between those aged sixteen or over who are or have been intimate partners or family members regardless of gender or sexuality (BWP, 2019).

Growing awareness of domestic violence

Awareness of the prevalence of domestic violence in our society is relatively recent. Social work textbooks published before 1970 featured detailed case analyses of individual interventions for different problematic situations, but domestic violence was not recognised as a social issue. A text book about social work relationships, published in the 1950s, described a woman telling a social worker that her husband 'knocked her about a bit but with no lasting damage'. This kind of statement evoked little reaction from the social work practitioners who read this and other similar accounts in the 1950s and 1960s. They were more concerned with the underlying psychodynamic relationships. Most professional practitioners lacked awareness of domestic violence. They tacitly accepted the legal and social *status quo* of the day, when married women had no legal rights to property of their own, were expected to give up their employment after marriage, were paid less, and divorce was very difficult to obtain.

Causes of domestic violence: feminist thinking and alternative theoretical explanations

The feminist movement in the 1960s promoted moves towards greater equality of the sexes and changed attitudes about male and female roles. Feminists drew attention to domestic violence against women and promoted views that domestic violence is prompted by men's traditional power over women. Programmes that were set up to offer support to abused women adopted this explanation, but other explanatory theories include *individualistic approaches* that locate the problem in the person, who has individual choices, characteristics, pathologies, and is capable of change; *familial and systems approaches*, that focus on family and couple interactions, and expect change to take place in all participants; *structuralist theories* (the approach adopted by feminists) that locate domestic violence in social, political, cultural and ideological structures rather than in individuals; a *social equality model of social change*, which identifies causal factors at different societal levels of violence – interpersonal, institutional, cultural and structural – with the remedy being to promote change at all levels; and *poststructuralist theories* that construct narratives about the reality of domestic violence (Scottish Government. Website accessed 12 March 2019).

George Monbiot, writing in the *Guardian* (16 January 2019) acknowledges that concepts of masculinity have changed, arguing that male protests about alleged threats to their identity are a sign of *fearful masculinity* triggered by anxiety about economic and national decline. *Fearful masculinity* then prompts some men to become misogynistic and homophobic as a way of countering their perceptions of diminishing power. Monbiot also argues against strength and aggressiveness being held up as the ideal of masculinity. He advocates that men should learn to acknowledge their weaknesses, share their personal fears, show concern for others, and not strive to prove their masculinity, instead, men can adopt 'emotional literacy and honest self-appraisal'.

The first women's refuge

In 1971, Erin Pizzey (born 1939) attracted publicity, support, and sufficient finance to establish Chiswick Women's Aid (now known as the charity Refuge) as the first refuge that offered a safe place where women whose partners had abused them could live free from victimisation. Pizzey encountered hostility from local residents as she expanded the number of shelters, but was also praised for setting up women's refuges at a time when most members of the public were not fully aware of the issues of domestic violence.

A number of charities now offer support to women and also men who experience domestic violence. Some of these organisations are national charities, for example, Refuge, Women's Aid, and the National Centre for Domestic Violence. Other charities are small, local organisations that offer different kinds of help to local women and men – supportive interventions that convey the message 'you are not alone'. The focus for many of the charities is on offering support to women who experience domestic violence.

> Practice Example 13.1: *Women's Work is a Derbyshire charity that provides confidential support to disadvantaged women and their families who are affected by domestic abuse, violence, drug and alcohol problems, homelessness and offending behaviours. Staff members offer confidential mentoring, family support, referrals to other relevant agencies, mediation, advocacy, direct access to drug treatment, counselling, advice on housing, benefits and budgeting and group and individual support.*

Theoretical influences: settlement houses, social pedagogy, and group care practice

Domestic violence charities communicate therapeutically by offering group work, individual support, short courses, and recreational activities to victims of abuse, an approach which is reminiscent of the support that settlement houses like Toynbee Hall (Briggs and Macartney, 2012) in London and Hull House in Chicago (Addams, 1935) offered to poor families in the late nineteenth and early twentieth centuries. Some helping strategies resemble aspects of social pedagogy (discussed in Chapter 17), for example, offering creative and group activities as therapy.

Theoretically, these charities' interventions also draw on aspects of the *group care practice model* developed by Ainsworth et al. (CCETSW, 1983). Group care practice promotes eight areas of knowledge and skills which illuminate how a group can be a therapeutic resource for communication:

1   *Organisation of the group care environment*, where practitioners understand and work within agreed organisational objectives, purposes, policies, and team structures, and use physical space and available equipment to create a positive atmosphere.
2   *Team functioning*, where practitioners collaborate with colleagues, and practice as a team member making positive contributions.
3   *Activity programming – educational, recreational, and free time*, where practitioners provide varied and new experiences, and share experiences and feelings in ways that promote positive attitudes and good feelings.
4   *Working with groups*, where practitioners plan and offer groups for learning, recreational or educational purposes, delivered with appropriate group intervention skills.
5   *On-the-spot counselling* (also discussed in Chapter 6) where practitioners make use of naturally occurring opportunities for counselling both purposefully and skilfully, without unduly disrupting planned programmes.
6   *Use of everyday life events*, where practitioners offer nurturing care, bodily comfort, and personal space that support efforts to modify attitudes and behaviours.
7   *Developmental scheduling*, where practitioners devise detailed care plans that recognise a person's individuality, for example, celebrating birthdays.
8   *Formulation of individual care and treatment plans* where practitioners keep a balance between individual and group needs, while providing satisfying individual experiences.

The Freedom Programme

In 2008, Pat Craven, a former social worker and probation officer who worked with male perpetrators, published a book, *Living with the Dominator*, which described the Freedom Programme. She devised this training programme in 1999 to communicate with women who were victims of domestic violence. Her goal was to help them better understand their situation, avoid blaming themselves, realise that they were not alone, and gain support. She rejected the reasons male perpetrators gave to explain their violence towards women (alcohol, low self-esteem, overwork, stress, joblessness), and argued that the cause is their desire to control women. The inspiration for her 'Dominator' concept is attributed to the Duluth Domestic Violence Intervention Project in Minnesota (Shepard and Pence, 1999).

The Dominator is portrayed as a

- *bully* who intimidates
- *headworker* who uses emotional abuse to destroy confidence
- *jailer* who isolates
- *liar* who makes false excuses
- *badfather* who uses children to gain control
- *King of the Castle* who treats his partner as a servant
- *sexual controller* who uses sex for control
- *persuader* who threatens and coerces

Craven attributes the prevalence of violence to the influence of traditional societal and cultural beliefs about male and female roles. She contrasts the 'Dominator's' characteristics with the qualities of a prototype 'Mr Right', a non-abusive man. She also compares each of the Dominator's qualities with the characteristics of a 'Friend', 'Goodfather', 'Confidence Booster', 'Liberator', 'Lover', 'Partner', 'Truthteller', and 'Negotiator'. She concludes the book with a list of helpful resources and suggestions for spotting a potential Dominator. Her training programme provides some easily grasped concepts and is widely used across the country as a supportive group programme for female victims of abuse.

Growing awareness that men experience domestic violence

As feminist thinking about male power began to challenge dominant societal attitudes about the roles of men and women, public awareness of domestic violence against women become widespread. Refuges and centres were set up to help women who experienced violence. Questions began to be asked about the now discredited belief that domestic violence is exclusively inflicted on women by male perpetrators. Domestic violence is now acknowledged to affect men as well as women. The facts and statistics about violence inflicted by women on men by were not recognised or acknowledged until relatively recently. Recognition that some women abuse their male partners increased. Erin Pizzey, who established the first women's refuge, supported this view. Her claim that women are also perpetrators of violence was unpopular amongst feminists, which may explain why her name tends not to be mentioned on the website of the organisation she founded. Pizzey did not portray men as the enemy; she thought that the childhood experience of growing up in an abusive home was a cause of domestic violence. Philip W. Cook, an American journalist, has written about women's abuse of men. Like Pizzey, he believes that childhood environments are causal factors of the abuse (Cook, 2009).

Signs that a man may be experiencing domestic violence include:

- fear and anxiety to please their partner
- going along with everything their partner says and does
- belittlement and verbal abuse
- low self-esteem
- fear they may lose their children
- health problems
- increased drinking or use of drugs
- increased isolation from friends and wider family

Suggestions for giving advice to a potential male survivor are similar to the suggestions offered to women survivors: express concern, offer acceptance, and believe what the victim is saying to you (Mankind Initiative, 2019).

What help is available for male survivors of domestic violence? Some charities focus on helping men escape domestic abuse situations, but these are few in number compared to the numbers of organisations that help women survivors.

- Women's Aid offers advice and information to male survivors.
- Survivors UK in London offers individual counselling (Survivors UK, 2019), group work and helpline services for individuals affected by male sexual violation.
- The Mankind Initiative, established in 2001 and based in Taunton, provides a helpline, a website that features survivors' stories, training and support for professional practitioners (including the police and local authorities), and information and advice for survivors (Mankind Initiative, 2019).
- The Public Health England Employers Toolkit provides information for employers who suspect one of their male employees may be experiencing abuse (PHE, 2019).

Programmes that attempt to bring about changes in perpetrators' behaviour

The main focus of domestic violence programmes is to provide help and support for survivors. What about the abusers who use violence and non-physical abuse to maintain control? Is it possible for them to learn how to stop their abusive behaviour? Can perpetrators of violence be helped to change? The answer is a qualified 'yes', although evidence of success is harder to verify because of fewer numbers coming forward, fewer programmes for perpetrators, and less research evidence.

Practice Example 13.2: *The Strength to Change Programme (Stanley et al., 2009; Stanley et al., 2011) is an NHS service for male perpetrators of domestic violence that began in 2009 in Hull. The NHS Hull service emphasises perpetrators' responsibilities for the abuse, is non-judgemental, and acknowledges perpetrators' ability to change their behaviours, and improve their own self-worth. The programme uses active listening, empathetic facilitation, non-judgemental attitudes, and non-*

acceptance of any form of abuse. 'Graduates' of the programmes are invited to help with group facilitation. The programme uses social marketing to attract individuals to the programme. Participants have reported that they developed more awareness of emotions, more self-control, more sensitivity to others' needs, and more self-esteem.

An example from Philadelphia, PA is an attempt to understand the motivations of male perpetrators.

Practice Example 13.3: Carrie Askin, a clinical social worker and therapist who is co-director of Menergy, a treatment programme in Philadelphia for emotionally and physically abusive partners, offers five reasons why some partners become abusive (Askin, 2015). These are: (1) difficulty tolerating emotional injury to one's self – blaming and retaliating when their feelings are hurt; (2) entitlement – believing they have a right not to be hurt or embarrassed, and punishing their partner when their entitlement is threatened; (3) lack of empathy – believing the other person wants to harm them, rather than being able to draw on emotional insight and understanding; (4) lack of accountability – believing that inflicting violence is acceptable; (5) hidden trauma – childhood experiences of abuse that may have 'normalised' the act of inflicting abuse.

Another example explains a therapist's approach with perpetrators:

Practice Example 13. 4: John G. Taylor, an Afro-American counsellor/therapist, offers help to men and women in abusive relationships. He provides group programmes that teach conflict resolution, negotiation, coping skills, respect, coping and communication skills, fairness, and exploration of the emotional effects their behaviours have on them and their partners. He believes that group therapy is important because it allows a perpetrator to be confronted by their peers and be held accountable. Individual therapy is also offered. Taylor concentrates on individual choices to be violent or not. He examines the roles that beliefs and assumptions about race, class, gender, religion, and sexual orientation and social, economic and environmental pressures play in the incidence of domestic violence (Taylor, 2019; Taylor, 2013).

More knowledge about the motivations that prompt perpetrators' actions and more knowledge about how to help perpetrators change their behaviours will further enable survivors of domestic violence gain help.

Domestic Violence bill

In January 2019, the British government published a draft Domestic Abuse bill designed to support victims and their families and pursue offenders. Along with this, the Home Office published a report on the economic and social costs of domestic abuse, which cost England and Wales £66 billion in 2016–17. This sum includes the costs of physical and emotional abuse on victims, and health, police, and victim services. The 'landmark bill' will introduce a statutory government definition of domestic abuse that includes economic abuse and controlling, manipulative non-physical abuse; a new role, the Domestic

Abuse Commissioner, to lead the responses to abuse issues; Domestic Abuse Protection Notices and Domestic Abuse Protection Orders to protect victims, including children; prohibit court cross-examination of victims by their abusers; provide automatic eligibility for special measures to support more victims to give evidence in criminal courts; and additional funding for disabled, elderly, and LGBT victims (Gov. UK, 2019 https://www..gov.uk/).

Charities have welcomed the bill on the whole, but pointed out gaps in support for migrant and asylum seekers who experience domestic abuse because they would risk deportation if they reveal the abuse (*Guardian*, 27 January 2019, https://www.theguardian.com/society/2019/ja/27).

Communicating with individuals who experience domestic violence

The first part of this chapter offered specific knowledge and theories about domestic violence as a necessary precursor for preparing practitioners to offer effective communication with survivors. Practitioners should familiarise themselves with the social contexts and underlying historical influences that are likely to trigger domestic violence. The impact of domestic violence may cause a person who is experiencing violence to 'freeze', panic, and be mistrustful.

Practice Example 13.5 *A middle-aged woman who had separated from her abusive partner became devastated and fearful when she thought about her previous contact with him. It was as if there were two persons sitting in the room: a capable intelligent woman who was a loving mother and grandmother, who had carried out a responsible job in which she supervised staff, and at the next moment when she thought about her ex-partner, a trembling frightened devastated individual who wrongly blamed herself for everything that had gone wrong.*

Communication with a frightened individual is not easy. Communication within groups can break down barriers of mistrust, and mend lack of confidence. One-to-one discussions with a professional practitioner must be honest about the extent of the practitioner's power and authority over the abused individual and about the extent and limitations of confidentiality if a person in the survivor's life continues to be abused.

Practice Example 13. *A young woman whose parents were dead and whose childhood included periods in local authority care, was successfully bringing up her children and staying away from drugs. She did not remember many details of her earlier life. She wanted to obtain the social services department's records of her time in care. She hoped to find proof that she had been sexually abused by a male relative, an action that her family always denied. She felt angry and let down, and wanted to find out more about what had happened to her.*

When listening to women who have experienced domestic abuse, a professional practitioner may discover an unacknowledged hidden childhood incident of sexual abuse committed by a family member, which damaged self-belief and esteem. Sometimes an abused woman may experience abuse from another member of the family – a brother, grandparent, or mother. Every account of abuse is different.

If someone you know tells you in confidence that they are experiencing domestic violence, your response is important. You will want to offer support and build trust. How can you do this?

- Proceed at a slow pace.
- Do not ask why the person doesn't leave the abuser, because leaving takes more courage than an abused person initially will have. The abused person probably will be fearful and isolated, with dependent children, little money, and nowhere to go.
- Listen to the victim's story without criticising or being judgemental.
- Accept that the story is truthful, even if your first instinct is shock and disbelief.
- Encourage the person to tell you how they feel. If they seem confused about their feelings for the abuser – both loving and fearing them – accept the feelings without accepting the violence.
- Give acceptance to the person who has just confided in you.
- Express concern for the person's safety.
- Offer to find out and share information about shelters, help lines, lawyers, refuges, and charities that can provide help and support, but recognise that it takes time for a survivor of domestic abuse to find the courage to walk away from an abusive situation.
- Continue to provide support and understanding.
- Avoid blaming or pressuring the survivor to leave, criticising or provoking the abuser, promising to help with something that you are not able to do, and ignoring the possibility of provoking physical danger.
- Help the person to make a safety plan before they take steps to leave (Very Well Mind, 2019).

Ongoing communication with survivors of domestic violence

Domestic violence can continue for years before a survivor seeks help. Restoring self-belief, self-confidence, and trust takes considerable time. The use of different supportive approaches, including educational and recreational group work, can help an individual feel safe and begin to look to the future. A person-centred approach (Rogers, 1961) that seeks to restore self-belief can be effective, and also a constructive approach (Neimeyer, 2009) that compliments the survivor on their good qualities and praises their unacknowledged strengths. Cognitive behaviour therapy and mindfulness may also be helpful on the journey to recovering belief in self.

References

Addams, J. (1935) *Forty Years at Hull House*. Macmillan: New York.

Askin, Carrie (2015) 'Five Reasons People Abuse Their Partners'. *Psychology Today*, 27 October 2015. https://www.psychologytoday.com. Website accessed 15 March 2019.

Briggs, A. and Macartney, A. (2012) *Toynbee Hall: The First Hundred Years*. Routledge: London (Routledge Revivals).

Broxtowe Women's Project (2019) *About Domestic Abuse.* https://broxtowewomensproject.org.uk Website accessed 8 March 2019.

CCETSW (Central Council for Education and Training in Social Work) (1983) *A Practice Curriculum for Group Care. Staff Development in the Social Services.* CCETSW Paper 14.2 CCETSW: London.

Cook, Philip W. (1997, 2009) *Abused Men: The Hidden Side of Domestic Violence.* Praeger ABC–CLIO: Santa Barbara, CA.

Craven, Pat (2008) *Living with the Dominator A book about the Freedom Programme.* Freedom Publishing: Knighton.

Gov.UK, (2019) 'Government publishes landmark domestic abuse bill', https://www..gov.uk/ 21 January 2019. Website accessed 10 March 2019.

Guardian (2019) 'Major gaps and missteps in domestic abuse bill', 27 January 2019, https://www.theguardian.com/society/2019/ja/27.

Mens Advice Line (2019). www.mensadviceline.org.uk Website accessed 13 March 2019.

Monbiot, George (2019) 'Why the men who assert their masculinity are stalked by fear', *The Guardian*, 16 January 2018, p. 3.

Neimeyer, R. A. (2009) *Constructivist Psychotherapy.* Routledge: London.

Pizzey, Erin and Shapiro, Jeff (1982) *Prone to Violence.* Hamlyn: London.

Refuge (2019) https://www.refuge.org.uk/ Website accessed 10 March 2019.

Public Health England (2019) *Domestic Violence Employers Toolkit.* www.wellbeing.bitc.org.uk Website accessed 13 March 2019.

Rogers, Carl (1961) *On Becoming a Person.* Constable: London.

Scottish Government. (2019) *Theories used to explain male violence against women partners and ex-partners.* https://www2.gov.scot/resource/doc/925/0063072.pdf. Website accessed 12 March 2019.

Shepard, M. and Pence, E. (eds) (1999) *Coordinating Community Responses to Domestic Violence. Lessons from Duluth and Beyond.* Sage: London.

Stanley, N., Fell, B., Miller, P., Thomson, G., and Watson, J. (2009) *Men's talk: research to inform Hull's social marketing initiative on domestic violence.* University of Central Lancashire: Lancashire.

Stanley, N., Borthwick, R., Graham-Kevan, N. and Chamberlain, R. (2011) *An evaluation of a new initiative for male perpetrators of domestic violence.* University of Central Lancashire: Lancashire.

Survivors UK (2019) www.survivorsuk.org. Website accessed 10 March 2009.

Taylor, John G. (2013) 'Behind the Veil: Inside the Mind of Men "That Abuse" Domestic Violence and unmasking the terror of Dr. Jekyll and Mr. Hyde', *Psychology Today.* https://www.psychologytoday.com 5 February. Website accessed 15 March 2019.

Taylor, John G. (2019) m.johngtaylor.com Website accessed 14 March 2019.

The Mankind Initiative (2019) https://www.mankind.org.uk/ Website accessed 15 February 2019.

Very Well Mind (2019) *9 Tips on How to Help a Victim of Domestic Violence.* https://www.verywellmind.com/. Website accessed 11 March 2019.

Women's Aid (2019) https://www.womensaid.org.uk/. Website accessed 10 March 2019.

Chapter 14

Communication through life stories and biographies

The meaning of biography

A *biography* is the story of a life written by another person, and an *autobiography* is the self-constructed story of one's own life. A biography is more than a chronological account of events in a person's life: the story of a life contains emotions that range from joy to sadness. Individuals remember past events selectively; they tell their stories according to the significance of a particular event, the era in which the event took place, and how they want to be perceived.

Every biography tells the story of a life as an interpretation of events rather than as objective facts. For the most part, published biographies and autobiographies focus on well-known people whose lives helped to shape the eras in which they lived. But what about the life experiences of people who are not famous, who lived 'ordinary' lives? During the twentieth century, historians began to collect *oral histories* taken from a range of people so that they could capture the authentic life experiences of individuals who lived through particular historical eras. The invention of microphones, tape recorders, and video cameras made it possible to capture and preserve their stories. Studying these accounts helps us to understand the values, habits, and beliefs that dominated their lives at a particular moment in time. This is the oral tradition of storytelling – interpretations and personal recollections of life experiences – which preceded written language. The roles of the *bard, chronicler* of history, and *story teller* have contributed to our cultural histories. Their stories are cultural interpretations of events that seek to enhance the understanding of listeners.

Theoretical perspectives on biographical accounts

Storytelling is a powerful means of communication. In the example below, an ancient mythological story resonates with Sigmund Freud's psycho–social theories.

> Practice Example 16.1 *Freud (1924) drew on Greek mythology to explain his Oedipus complex which describes how a young child may feel desire for the parent of the opposite sex and jealousy towards the parent of the same sex. Oedipus was a character in Sophocles' play Oedipus Rex who kills his father by accident and subsequently unknowingly marries his mother. In the Greek myth, Oedipus was abandoned at birth and therefore did not know who his parents were. After he had killed his father and married his mother, he learns their true identities. Freud theorised that a boy may feel that he is competing with his father for possession of his mother, while a girl may feel that she must*

compete with her mother for her father's affections. According to Freud, children regard their same-sex parent as a rival for the opposite-sex parent's attention.

Although Freud's theories of psycho-social development (1986 editions) stop short of exploring development in adult life, the psychologist Erik Erikson (1950, 1986) argued that development continues throughout childhood and adult life as eight developmental crises that individuals can resolve by making choices towards either psycho-social growth or decline. The crises of infancy (with the choice of basic trust vs. basic mistrust), early childhood (autonomy vs. shame, doubt), play age (initiative vs. guilt), school age (industry vs. inferiority), adolescence (identity vs. confusion), young adulthood (intimacy vs. isolation), adulthood (generativity vs. self-absorption) and old age (integrity vs. despair) set out the choices that individuals must make at each stage of their development. The stages are presented in an orderly sequence that Erikson et al. (1986) called *epigenetic*. The way each crisis is resolved lays the groundwork for resolving the next crisis. The ways that we use biographical methods – telling stories and explaining significant events in our lives – as part of our communication with each other suggest that development is possible in adult life, and as such, our biographical accounts reflect the influence of Erikson's theories that allow for changes in adult life, thus reducing feelings of despair and hopelessness.

The autobiographical stories that we tell about ourselves are not fixed entities, but may change and develop over time as we make connexions between present and past, and explore issues of how past relationships may influence present relationships. As we develop throughout our life, we construct and reconstruct our beliefs. Individual well-being is influenced not only by emotions, feelings, inner drives and social and environmental factors, but also by the ways that people search for meaning through constructing ideas about the significance of particular events.

- Neimeyer (2009, discussed in Chapter 6) uses reconstructive theories and therapeutic techniques in his practice to help his patients develop new perspectives of their life situations.
- Viktor Frankl's logotherapy (1969, also discussed in Chapter 6) identifies the *search for meaning* as a significant motivating force for human behaviour, and encourages individuals to share their *personal narratives* as part of their search for meaning.

The biographical approach as a research technique

The biographical approach is used as a research technique as well as for therapeutic interventions. The biographical research technique links with the sociological theory of symbolic interactionism (Blumer, 1969). Symbolic interactionism focuses on meaning, language and thought as core principles for the development of the self, and explores individuals' interactions with each other, the symbolic meanings and subsequent behaviours derived from these interactions, and the shared understandings that arise from interpretations of the interactions.

Biographical research is qualitative research that uses observation and interviews to capture pictures of an individual's life events, values, and the meanings they give to their lives, but the contemporary demand for evidence-based practice favours quantitative methods like large-scale surveys rather than individual interviews. Qualitative research is usually small scale, exploratory, and used to develop ideas for further research. Quantitative research is large scale and uses numerical data and statistics to establish new, verifiable knowledge. Allen, Fairclough, and Heinzen (2002) argue that narratives contain emotions, that telling stories can help to explore different perspectives on issues, and that these stories enable hidden emotions to come to the surface. They suggest that story telling respects people and recognises complex relationships. Lieblich and Josselson (1997) affirm that life stories can help to construct individual identity, and criticise editors who change individual narratives. They identify two different approaches to gathering life stories: the *socio-cultural approach*, portraying how people live in communities; and the *sociolinguistic approach*, portraying an individual's search for identity. They compare the construction of a life story to an individual editing their curriculum vitae or choosing how to present themselves at a job interview.

Ethical issues

Interviewing individuals and listening to their life stories can pose ethical dilemmas when data is collected for research purposes and also for therapeutic purposes. The key question is: to whom does a collected life story belong? Who has the right to interpret the story, and publish the life story in publications, thus perhaps changing their intended meanings? Will the publication of biographical research and biographical material cause harm and offence to individuals who share details of their lives with a researcher or practitioner?

The potential for causing unwitting harm must not be overlooked. Practising within data protection legal requirements is an essential requirement. Every practitioner and researcher who uses biographical methods needs to abide by ethical guidelines. As a first step, it is important to build a trusting relationship with the individual who shares their life story. That trust should be maintained throughout an interview and afterwards, when decisions have to be made about how to use the collected data. Confidentiality must be preserved for individuals who share details of their lives. Before individuals agree to participate, they should be informed about safeguards to their confidentiality and the planned uses of the data.

The biographical approach as therapeutic communication

Establishing a personal identity is helped by an individual's personal interpretation of their life events that shapes their individual autobiography. Their individual interpretation of life can be constructive (Neimeyer, 2009) and lead to increased understanding and acceptance of the individual self. Alternatively, an interpretation can be destructive and self-punitive. Professional practitioners often listen to individuals who communicate despair. The act of telling their story to a sympathetic listening ear can help them understand previously chaotic life events. A constructive approach views the opportunity of sharing one's life story as a learning activity through which an individual can reconstruct or reinterpret the events of their life, and thus develop better self-understanding.

The Swiss psychologist, Jean Piaget (2013, 1999) developed constructivism as a philosophy of education that promotes educational techniques like learning by discovery – learning with and from one's peers rather than solely by teacher-led didactic instruction.

Constructive educational theory believes that individuals learn from making sense of how their life experiences and their own ideas and values interact. The leap from this educational constructivist philosophy to the social constructivist ideas that influence professional communication in health, social work and counselling is a logical step.

Do professional assessments fit with the biographical approach?

A professional practitioner may be required to complete an *assessment* of 'need' that gathers facts about an individual's situation and the reasons they ask for help. (Some, but not all aspects of an assessment might be described in health care practice as a *social history*.) An assessment helps to determine eligibility for, or fit with, the services that might be offered. An assessment usually requires completion of a pre-designed pro forma, which may detract from the process of developing constructive relationships. The practitioner whose eyes are fixed on the forms they have to complete, who rarely looks at the person sitting before them, and who moves purposefully and swiftly from one question to another in a business–like manner will not form a trusting relationship and may perhaps miss the realities of the person's situation. He or she will appear solely as an authority figure who communicates the minimum amount of empathy. Although an assessment has to gather some biographical details, the practitioner's communication style may overlook opportunities for using the assessment as constructive practice that explores the client's social reality.

Life story work with children and young people

Life story books are a kind of biographical technique which are used to prepare children and young people for permanency – usually adoption. Social workers who practise with children and young people want to help children in long-term foster care establish a sense of identity by learning more about their social, cultural and racial origins. The received wisdom is that the children's self-esteem will increase if they gain a fuller understanding of their own identity. Their early childhood years may have been disrupted by experiences of frequent moves, different caregivers, and the absence of their parents. Their memories of the changes in their lives, may not be understood, or might be forgotten. They may have no available written accounts of their early childhood – no pictures and no reminiscences. A life story book can help fill in the gaps and hopefully develop a stronger sense of identity.

Yet there are pitfalls. Is identity to be discovered through knowing about one's origins and heredity, or through constructive learning experiences arising from a child's environment? Our ability to use language for communicating with each other depends not only on intellectual abilities but on being given developmental opportunities to learn a language through listening to others' speech. The issue of identity is complex. Are we a product of our heredity or our environment, or both?

> Practice Example 16.2 *When I grew up in the USA in a suburban community seven miles from New York City, my classmates at school came from families with different national origins. Nearly all of us had parents or grandparents who had emigrated to the US from another country. We introduced ourselves by stating our names. We would then ask each other: 'what are you?' – and the answers*

> *would be 'Italian', 'Armenian', 'German', 'Polish', 'French', 'Hungarian', 'English' or 'Irish', etc. We knew that we were Americans but the word was hyphenated to reflect the national origin 'Italian-American', etc. However, the black children in the class were never asked about their origins; in that northern part of the US, the white children did not think about the history of slavery and segregation in the southern states. Perhaps because of the children's different backgrounds, their educational curriculum emphasised learning 'how to be' – using correct grammar, displaying good table manners, being polite, taking care of health, and eating a well-balanced diet, as well as learning about American history, were lessons aimed at helping the children construct their identities as Americans.*

Children and young people in care can be helped to build their identity and develop a sense of belonging by adopting a constructivist point of view that identity formation is an interactive process that blends an individual's social contexts and their individual thoughts and learning with how they make sense of their world. Identity is not irrevocably shaped by one's past. A life story can become a therapeutic tool when it is constructed collaboratively and empathetically, and sufficient time is given to discuss the issues that arise.

Undertaking life story work

A life story book is intended to prepare a child for a new permanent placement. The life story is a record of the child's life up to the placement – with pictures, facts, and stories and the reasons why they could not continue to live with their birth parents. The book is meant for the child. Because the life story has to include information of a sensitive nature (that some children are not able to live with their birth parents because of abuse or neglect), too fast a pace could be damaging. Ryan and Walker's *Life Story Work* (2016) asks practitioners to consider whether they are the right person to undertake this work, whether their agency is committed, and whether they will receive training and support, etc. (These questions are directed at the practitioner rather than at their employer.) Ryan and Walker advise practitioners to avoid clichés when talking to a child. Life story work can be undertaken digitally, and also can be used with children with a life-threatening illness. Importantly, they suggest that the life story work does not have to result in a 'product' – rather, it is the communication process that counts (p. 5).

> Practice Example 16.3: *A county council's published advice for social workers who undertake life story work with children contains over 200 separate 'dos and don'ts' arranged in a series of bullet points – in effect, the advice informs the social workers what to do without supplying adequate explanations of how to make a professional judgement or how much or how little information should be shared with the child. The advice states that the social workers are required to have regular professional supervision but gives no guarantees that their employer will undertake to offer this support.*

Life histories of adults

Adult life histories serve different purposes, ranging from family reminiscences at social occasions, to reminiscence therapy used with people with dementia, to a therapeutic intervention with a troubled individual. Accounts of remembered events in childhood delineate the interface between individual lives and historical changes.

> Practice Example 16.4 *An eighty-three-year-old man recalled a time during the Second World War when at the age of six, he travelled with his parents on the train to Manchester to spend Christmas with his grandparents in Lancashire. When they arrived, the family discovered the station had been bombed and was on fire. He remembers leaving the station, which was in chaos, with his parents and then walking with them through the city streets to the other railway station to catch their train to their final destination. He felt afraid and he realised that his parents were also frightened. His recollections formed a vivid part of his life history.*

Therapeutic use of life history work

Individuals who were abused in their childhood, or who led unsettled lives may benefit from participating in a collaborative process to share their life histories, ask questions, and reflect on what has happened to them over the years. The process of writing a short life story of an individual who seeks help can be an effective therapeutic tool. This is not the same as researching their lives as part of a research project.

First, the practitioner must gain the trust of the individual and discuss confidentiality and the purpose of the life history. One or two meetings between the individual and a professional practitioner provide occasions to discuss, consider, and select information to include in the life story – not only losses and tragedies, but also the happy moments of that life. When a person and a practitioner reach agreement about what will be included, a word processed biographical account of no more than two or three pages can be presented to the individual to keep. This process can enable an individual to identify positive attributes and happy moments as well as sad events, and allows constructive thinking about the self to take hold. The process cannot be rushed, and should allow for regular scrutiny and alterations to the history as it gradually unfolds.

A more elaborate version of the life history could contain pictures and important documents. Individuals who have experienced many changes and moves may not remember all the details of their past. Women who have been abused can benefit from constructing life histories that emphasise their strengths and resilience. A life history can capture significant moments and review past decisions, along with present-day reflections. Life stories that are anecdotally told can be negative, and convey impressions of being a 'bad seed' 'just like your father' or 'just like your mother', but these are deterministic histories that are imposed involuntarily on an individual. An authentic life history cannot be wholly defined entirely by an individual's heredity or family history, but by lived experiences and reflections. A life history belongs to the individual who tells his or her life story; professional practitioners should respect this, and not amend the life history of an individual unless the individual gives permission.

Narrative therapy

Narrative therapy (White and Epston, 1990; Morgan, 2000) suggests different uses of the biographical approach. Narrative therapy is a collaborative method that enables individuals to tell their own stories in the hope that they will begin to develop a more affirmative narrative about their lives. As such, narrative therapy is part of a constructivist view of identity. Narrative therapy seeks to concentrate on individual strengths, and emphasises the positive aspects of their individuality. This theoretical approach separates the *person* from the *problem*. (In this, narrative therapy resembles Perlman's 1957 classic problem-solving social work method which identified the *person*, the *problem*, and the *place* as separate key issues.) Narrative therapy views the *person* positively and assumes that he or she has the skills and expertise that will enable them to problem-solve and reconstruct their personal narratives towards a more positive view of themselves. The *problem* is externalised in narrative therapy, so the person no longer feels burdened with guilt and self-criticism.

Reminiscence therapy

Reminiscence therapy, another variation of biographical methods, is usually offered to groups of older people, including those with dementia. Robert Butler (1963) suggested that the technique of the life review could become a therapeutic support, rather than be seen as a sign of decline in old age. Reminiscence can help preserve living memories for others. Reminiscence therapy can take place in a group. Listening together to remembered songs helps to trigger memories. The use of artefacts from the past – old kitchen implements like a cheese grater or a coffeepot are not necessarily a spur to memory but are an affirmation of life experience and a boost to individual identity.

Specific examples of biographical approaches

Examples of the specific use of reminiscence, narrative and a biographic approach can be found in the collected stories, novels, and poetry about the experiences of Holocaust survivors who were Kindertransport children, photographic portrayals of displaced peoples around the world, the lives of refugees, and the experiences of the child migrants.

Stories of Holocaust survivors

During the Holocaust of the Second World War (1939–1945), between five and six million Jews, as well as seven million Russian, Polish and Yugoslav prisoners and civilians and thousands of gypsies and people with handicaps were murdered in concentration camps. Remembering and acknowledging the importance of the Holocaust is important for our collective understanding, before living memories of the Holocaust will vanish entirely. (The Holocaust Museum is recording some of these memories, so their testimonies can live on). In 2019, a *Guardian* article (Sherwood, 2019) stated that a poll commissioned by the Holocaust Memorial Day Trust revealed that one in twenty British adults does not believe or does not know that the Holocaust events ever happened. Half of those who were questioned did not know how many Jews were murdered, and markedly underestimated the numbers who were killed. These results were attributed largely to the people who were polled lacking knowledge, rather than being Holocaust deniers. This is why the stories of Holocaust survivors are a powerful communication.

Practice example 16.5 *The Holocaust Museum is located in peaceful countryside in Nottinghamshire, with a memorial garden, exhibitions, and displays about the Holocaust, including the story of a young boy sent to Britain by his parents to escape the Holocaust. Survivors give regular talks to audiences of children and families, and the Museum is recording their memories as a legacy for the future.*

Learning from the lives of the Kindertransport children

Practitioners can learn from the biographical accounts of children who came to Britain on the Kindertransport programme from Germany before the outbreak of the Second World War. Trainloads of over 9000 Jewish children were sent to Britain for refuge. Most of the children did not realise at the time that they would never see their parents again. Accounts of the lives of these children illustrate their resilience, but also provide understanding of what actually made a difference once they arrived in England.

The testimonies of survivors and survivors' children can help professional practitioners understand the children's responses to their lack of knowledge about what happened to their parents, and being placed in foster homes and hostels. These life stories and reflections can teach practitioners much about issues for practice: how the children searched for knowledge and understanding of why their lives were disrupted, and what had happened to their parents. Some themes reflect current practice issues: life story work, support for loss, the need for attachment, and resilience.

- The novelist Penelope Lively wrote an autobiographical account (2001) of her youth during the Second World War, in which she portrayed the helping activity of her aunt who worked as a volunteer, resettling refugees, including some Kindertransport children.
- The parents of David Attenborough, the broadcaster and naturalist, and Richard Attenborough, the actor, fostered two Jewish sisters who were refugees from Germany for seven years, and the brothers kept in touch with the sisters throughout their lives.

When they reached adulthood, some Kindertransport children wrote biographical accounts about the Kindertransport. Karen Gershon (1966) collected the life stories of the children who had travelled to Britain on the Kindertransport trains. These experiences impacted on their identities. The reader learns about their individual struggles and adaptation. Themes expressed in Gershon's collection of narratives include:

- recollections of the moment of leaving their parents
- becoming a refugee
- their gradual realisations that their parents were dead
- confusion about their own identities, perceiving themselves as German, Jewish, and without roots
- feelings in adulthood, for some, that they had become a part of a community

Bertha Leverton and Schmul Lowehnsohn (1990) presented first-hand reminiscences by the Kindertransport children, made when they were in late adulthood. The older children fared less well than the younger ones. They had to fend for themselves very soon after arriving; they were placed in hostels and had to find work, and then were interned as enemy aliens at the outbreak of war. The younger children were placed in foster homes which varied in quality. Most of their parents died in the concentration camps, but a few parents did survive, and in some instances, relationships between a reunited parent and their child became stressful after the years spent apart, perhaps due to unrecognised traumatic stress. Some children remained in the United Kingdom, others emigrated to the USA and Israel as they grew older.

Children of the survivors

The Kindertransport children are now in their late adulthood and some have died of old age. The life experiences of some of these Holocaust survivors have been told in auto-biographical accounts (Fremont, 1999; Epstein, 1997; Pilcer, 2001) written by their own adult children who grew up in Britain or the USA. Their stories reveal the impact of the separation and their lack of knowledge of what had happened to their parents.

> Practice Example 16.6 *When I presented a paper at an international conference, I met two adult children of Holocaust survivors. They came forward to talk to me privately, prompted by my brief mention of the Kindertransport in my paper. One woman worked for a charity that helped refugees; the other worked for an international agency in Bangladesh. Both women affirmed the influence on their own lives of their mothers' experiences as Holocaust survivors.*

Poetry as story telling

Lotte Kramer (1994a, 1994b, 1997) came to Britain on the last Kindertransport train in 1939. She published several volumes of evocative poetry that reflects on her refugee experience, identity, history, and relationships. The poem below portrays her search for her lost parents:

> *Searching for parents (Kramer, 1997, Selected and New Poems 1980–1997, p. 83)*
>
> Then I'd rush home at night and look for a mail
>
> From Europe, via the Red Cross, maybe,
>
> To say my parents had been traced, though frail
>
> And ill but still alive...a dream for me
>
> And many others. A sterile make-believe
>
> That led to nightmares, split my mind. The days
>
> Were filled with slogging work. I buried grief,
>
> Hunter for rations, joined banana queues.
>
> Now looking back from years they never reached

> I wonder who she was, this person 'I'
>
> Who rushed up the bare stair-boards that we shared
>
> With other tenants in the house. I try
>
> Pursuing her into our two room flat
>
> And will not find that letter on the mat.

Search for identity: Sebald's novel *Austerlitz*

W.G. Sebald (1944–2002) wrote the novel *Austerlitz* (2001) about Jacques Austerlitz, a lecturer in architectural history at a London institute of art history, who tells his life story to a confidante in a series of meetings from 1967 to 1996. Gradually, in retirement, Austerlitz begins to confront his repressed memories of his early childhood identity. His seemingly unconnected reflections to his confidante on railway station architecture, clocks and time, railway journeys, the flight of homing pigeons, moths and butterflies, airplanes, and the architecture of fortresses are revealed as the traces of his childhood memory when he was parted in 1939 at the age of five from his Jewish parents in Prague and travelled on a Kindertransport train to England. He was placed with Welsh foster parents who provided shelter and an education but no love and affection. Austerlitz' lack of love in his foster home is not noticed. Knowledge of his earlier identity is denied him, and his foster parents die without providing any information about his origins.

He grows up without being given any information about his early identity. In late middle age, he determines to find out the identity of his parents and what happened to them. He begins to piece together his fragments of memory. For the first time in his consciousness, he confronts the horror of the systemic Nazi war machine and the realities of the Holocaust. He learns that his mother was sent to Terezin concentration camp, while his father was away in Paris. When Austerlitz embarks on his journey of discovery he is approaching middle age. At the end of the novel he is old, yet still searching to develop his sense of self in old age.

Displaced people: communicating life stories through photographic images

Photographic images can communicate the lives of people in different cultures and situations. The Brazilian–born photographer and former economist Sebastiao Salgado recorded the relocation of people who were displaced because of war, famine, and economic globalisation. He photographed war refugees in Africa, Asia, and the Balkans, and in Asia and Latin America, people seeking work who moved from rural areas to crowded fast-growing cities. His book *Migrations* (2001) contains, inter alia, photographs of refugees from Kabul in Afghanistan (p. 83), Croatian refugees living on a chicken farm (p. 125), gypsies from Kosovo (pp. 150–151), orphans in Zaire waiting for food that never comes (p. 213), and abandoned babies in Sao Paulo, Brazil (pp. 314–315).

The stories of asylum-seeking refugees

The presence of asylum-seeking families and unaccompanied refugee children in the United Kingdom raises contemporary issues for human rights. Their biographical stories echo the historic accounts of the Kindertransport children. In 2019, the Refugee Council's Children's Section featured stories of child refugees on its website (https://www.refugeecouncil.org.uk/animation, accessed 30 January 2019):

- ML arrived in the UK when she was 12, sent alone from Nigeria to live with a family friend. She lived as a domestic servant, and was beaten and sexually abused.
- MT escaped from the Taliban in Afghanistan at the age of 15, and reached the UK after a dangerous three-month journey.
- F left Afghanistan when he was 15. After reaching the UK, he was held in a detention centre as an adult because the authorities did not believe he was a child.

Selam Kidane's website (https://selamkidanedotcom.wordpress.com/, accessed 31 January 2019) uses poetry and short accounts to continue to build public awareness of refugees. These issues are not new. In 2001, Kidane, an Eritrean psychotherapist, writer, and human rights campaigner who was herself an asylum seeker, published stories of unaccompanied children who sought asylum:

- A, aged 15, from Afghanistan: *If I could go back home I would …I have no home to go back to and every time you see something on the news and people look at you in a different way, you just know that they don't trust you, they don't believe you and they do not understand about you.*
- A, aged 17, from Ethiopia: *I want people to understand the pain of being alone.*
- S, aged 15, from Somalia: *In the refugee camp I was too worried about my family to play with the other children.*

Learning from historic practice: stories of the child migrants

Child migration (Humphries, 1994; Bean and Melville, 1989) was a British government policy that sent children in care from the United Kingdom to live in other countries (Australia, New Zealand, Canada), without the permission of their parents. The policy separated the children from their country of origin, removed any possibility of reunification with parents, and denied children their own personal histories and identities. The independent Nottingham–based Child Migrant Trust, headed by Margaret Humphreys, has told the stories of the child migrants. In 2010, a film called *Oranges and Sunshine* was made about her work.

Child migration was mainly carried out by voluntary agencies whilst the statutory child care service focused on closing down institutions and introducing rehabilitative programmes for children. Child migration was allowed to continue until 1967, and contemporary professional child care texts written in the 1960s (Stroud, 1965; Kastell, 1962; ACCO, 1964) which sought to promote higher social work standards did not mention child migration's continuing existence. Professional practitioners may question why child migration continued for so long. The belief that emigration offered a better life contradicted the known evidence of Bowlby's attachment theory (1951).

Developing *empathetic snapshots*

Professional communication sometimes fails to convey empathy. Because professional practitioners face conflicting demands and are sometimes required to work in a process-oriented manner, consequently they may not be able to respond with empathy to the situations of those they are trying to help. Professional practitioners can develop empathy by drawing on person-centred theory (Rogers, 1961) and biographical vignettes to form *empathetic snapshots* that illuminate understanding, and enable them to transfer their empathetic understanding from one situation to another.

Practice Example 16.7 *During Holocaust week, Fiona Boyd, a social worker who teaches at the University of Derby, attended a lecture given by a woman who had come to Britain as a child in the Kindertransport. Touched by the account of children leaving their parents and families and coming on their own from Germany to Britain, Fiona asked the woman if she had any relevant messages for social workers working with children from asylum-seeking families. She gave Fiona two very strong messages: first, the children's need to belong; and second, social workers need continually to question and examine their roles within a state-led system. The woman's messages and her account of her childhood experiences formed an empathetic snapshot that led Fiona to seek a deeper understanding of children within asylum-seeking families.*

Some concluding thoughts

This chapter has discussed communication that uses **life stories** and **biographical approaches** as a research method and a therapeutic technique. Life stories and biographical approaches can be a therapeutic tool for practice with children and adults who have experienced turbulent lives, if the life stories are constructed collaboratively within an atmosphere of trust and confidentiality. Every individual develops certain beliefs – 'constructions' about themselves and the events in their lives – and a biographical approach can help them reach new understandings. Finally, it must be reiterated that professional practitioners who use life story work and other biographical techniques in their practice must possess appropriate skills, receive skilled and regular practice supervision, and systematically review the ethical issues of practice decisions. Communicating with life stories and biographical techniques helps to build empathy and understanding, and enables individuals' voices to be heard.

References

ACCO Association of Child Care Officers (1964) *The Duties and Functions of Child Care Officers.* ACCO: London.

Allen, Jill, Fairclough, Gerald, and Heinzen, Barbara (2002) *The Power of the Tale. Using Narratives for Organisational Success.* John Wiley & Sons: Chichester, West Sussex.

Bean, P. and Melville, J. (1989) *Lost Children of the Empire. The Untold Story of Britain's Child Migrants.* Unwin Hyman: London.

Blumer, Herbert (1969) *Symbolic Interactionism: Perspective and Method.* Prentice Hall: Englewood Cliffs, NJ.

Bowlby, John (1951). *Maternal care and mental health*. World Health Organization Monograph. New York.

Butler, Robert N. (1963) 'The Life Review: An Interpretation of Reminiscence in the Aged' *Psychiatry. Interpersonal and Biological Processes*. Volume 26, Issue 1, pp. 65–76.

Epstein, Helen (1997) *Where She Came From. A Daughter's Search for Her Mother's History*. Plume: New York.

Erikson, E. (1950, 1986) *Childhood and Society*. WW Norton: New York.

Erikson, E., Erikson, J. and Quivnick, H. (1986) *Vital Involvement in Old Age*. WW Norton: New York.

Frankl, V. (1969) *Man's Search for Ultimate Meaning*. Basic Books: Cambridge, MA.

Fremont, Helen (1999) *After Long Silence. A memoir*. Delta: New York.

Freud, S. (1924, 1961) 'The dissolution of the Oedipus complex'. *The standard edition of the complete psychological works of Sigmund Freud: Vol.19 (1923–1925), Ego and the id, and other works*. Hogarth Press and the Institute of Psychoanalysis: London, pp. 172–179.

Freud, S. (1986 edition) *The Essentials of Psycho-Analysis* (selected by Anna Freud). Penguin: London.

Gershon, Karen (ed.) (1966) *We Came As Children. A Collective Autobiography of Refugees*. Gollancz: London.

Humphries, Margaret (1994) *Empty Cradles*. Doubleday: London.

Kastell, Jean (1962) *Casework in Child Care*. Routledge, Kegan Paul: London.

Kidane, Selam (2001) *I did not choose to come here. Listening to refugee children*. BAAF: London.

Kramer, Lotte (1994) 'The Ladder', *The Desecration of Trees*. Hippopotamus Press: Frome, Somerset, p. 25.

Kramer, Lotte (1994) *Earthquake and Other Poems*. Rockingham Press, Ware: Hertfordshire.

Kramer, Lotte (1997) *Selected and New Poems 1980–1997*. Rockingham Press in association with the European Jewish Publication Society: Ware, p. 85.

Leverton, Bertha and Lowensohn, Shmuel, eds. (1990) *I Came Alone. The Stories of the Kindertransports*. The Book Guild Ltd.: Sussex.

Lieblich, Amia, and Josselson, Ruthellen, eds. (1997) *The Narrative Study of Lives*. Volume 5. Sage: London.

Lively, Penelope (2001) *A House Unlocked*. Penguin: London.

McLeod, John (1997) *Narrative and Psychotherapy*. Sage: London.

Morgan, Alice (2000) *What is narrative therapy? An easy-to-read introduction*. Gecko Press: Wellington, NZ.

Neimeyer, R. (2009) *Constructivist Psychotherapy*. Routledge: London.

Oppenheimer, Deborah, and Harris, Mark Jonathan (2008)*Into the Arms of Strangers: Stories of the Kindertransport*. Bloomsbury/St Martins: New York & London.

Perlman, H. H. (1957). *Social Casework: A Problem Solving Process*. The University of Chicago: Chicago.

Piaget, J. (2013, 1999) *The Construction of Reality in the Child* (Volume 82). Routledge: London.

Pilcer, Sonia (2001) *The Holocaust Kid*. Delta: New York.

Rogers, Carl (1961) *On Becoming a Person: a Therapist's View of Psychotherapy*. Constable: London.

Ryan, T. and Walker, R. (2016) *Life Story Work: A Practical Guide to Helping Children Understand Their Past*. BAAF (British Association for Adoption and Fostering): London.

Salgado, Sebastiao (2001) *Migrations: Humanity in Transition*. Amazonas Images, Aperture Foundation: New York

Sebald, W. G. (2001) *Austerlitz*. Translated from German by Anthea Bell. Hamish Hamilton: London.

Sherwood, Harriet (2019) 'One in 20 Britons say the Holocaust never happened, shock poll finds', *The Guardian*, 27 January 2019, p. 9.

Stroud, J. (1965*) An Introduction to the Child Care Service*. Longmans: London.

White, M. and Epston, D. (1990) *Narrative Means to Therapeutic Ends*. W. W. Norton: New York.

Communicating with older people

How are older people perceived?

Chapter 15 begins with questions:

- How do you, as a practitioner, communicate with an old person?
- Do you think of older people as a group set apart from the rest of humanity because they are old?
- Do you sometimes try to avoid old people because their appearance triggers unwelcome thoughts about your own journey towards old age and eventual death?

These are questions to ask yourself when you practise with older people. You may want to take a few minutes to reflect on your response to these questions. If you find yourself slipping into involuntary thoughts about older people being difficult to deal with, then it is time to reconsider how you think about people who are old. Peter Townsend (1958), a famous researcher of older people's lives, admitted his unease and lack of confidence when he began to interview older people. Rather than drawing on pre-conceived negative ideas about older people, professional practitioners will benefit from learning what older people are really like.

Stereotyping older people

The press, the media, and considerable numbers of people sometimes stereotype older people as pathetic, confused, out of touch and incapable. They may unwittingly use prejudicial language when speaking directly to an older person or when they talk about older people in conversation with their colleagues. This kind of communication belittles older people.

Practice Example 15.1: Some people address old people as if they were speaking to a young child, by using overly familiar diminutives – 'dear', 'my darling', 'my lovely', or they may refer to older individuals as 'the elderly' (not as people), or as 'OAPs' (old age pensioners), 'old geezers', 'old buffers', or 'grandma' or 'grandpa'. Some individuals tell everyone who reaches retirement age to 'just put your feet up' and thus discourage them from taking up new activities. This kind of language and behaviour demeans older people rather than allowing them to be recognised as individuals.

Another reaction, intended to show concern but which becomes patronising instead, is when a professional practitioner suddenly softens their voice and addresses a bereaved older person in a manner meant to show concern, but which fails to disguise the practitioner's underlying unease: *'are you all right?'* Sometimes a practitioner asks in a hushed tone: *'how are you?'* The voice drips with concern, but also signals the practitioner's dread and anxiety. The practitioner can barely conceal their relief when the older person replies *'I'm fine'*, allowing the practitioner to rapidly change the subject and talk about more inconsequential matters. Unfortunately the older person may recognise the practitioner's unease and then decide to avoid talking about their true feelings, thus 'saving' the practitioner. Is this good communication?

When does old age begin?

When do people become old? This is a more complicated question than one might first think. If you believe that old age begins when a person becomes eligible to draw their pension, then you soon have to acknowledge that government decisions can change the ages when a person can draw their state pension. In the UK, pension ages for men and women used to differ – 65 years for men and 60 years for women. Since 2010, the pension age for women has risen and will be set at 65 years by 2010, and then will rise to 66, 67 and 68 years for both men and women, a move prompted by increases in longevity. Along with this change, the previous convention of setting a compulsory retirement age has been abolished, so people who are eligible to draw their state pension can continue working if they wish (The Pensions Advisory Service, 2019).

Alternatively, should a person be designated as 'old' when they develop a chronic debilitating physical and mental condition and no longer consider themselves to be in good health? Some younger people, as well as older people, may develop disabling conditions. Considerable numbers of older people retain their good health and largely avoid the experience of severe aches and pains when they reach their sixties and seventies (WHO, 2014). Does society consider a person 'old' when their hair turns grey and wrinkles appear on their face, even though their intellectual abilities and personalities are not affected? These issues give rise to uncertainty about when old age begins and what it means, and hopefully the uncertainty will prompt new kinds of thinking about old age.

Different experiences of old age

Some older people look forward to retirement and others dread it. Four factors make a difference to a person's attitude to retirement: the amount of money they have, their health, whether they are able to enjoy a range of leisure interests, and whether they can maintain satisfying relationships with friends and family (WHO, 2011). In contrast, older persons who have little income to look forward to when retired, who have major debts, no close family, and who live in unsatisfactory accommodation or who are homeless may not be able to enjoy retirement. *Intersectionality* (Collins and Bilge, 2016, discussed in Chapter 2) influences individual experiences of old age, with older women of colour likely to be less well off than older men, thus facing the *triple jeopardy* of age, gender, and race (Phillips, Ajrouch, and Hillcoat-Nalletanby, 2010). Older persons who maintain a network of satisfying relationships, despite lack of money and poor health, are more likely to enjoy a happy old age.

Practice Example 15.2 *Mr. P. and Mrs. S., who both live in an old people's home, spent every afternoon together, sitting and talking about their interest in the countryside and wild life. Mr. P. had worked as a farm labourer and had never married. Mrs. S. was a widow who had loved gardening. At first glance they seemed to have little in common because of the differences in their education and life styles, but they formed a satisfying friendship based on their mutual interests.*

Healthy ageing and activities

Age UK and NHS England promote the concept of *healthy ageing* (2015) – and that means eating nutritious food, not over-eating, exercising regularly, and avoiding excessive drinking or drug taking, as well as monitoring blood pressure and other health indicators. The NHS public health initiative (HM Government, 2010) urges older people to adopt a healthy life style in old age, but not everyone chooses to follow a healthy life style. Many older people may be unaware of what 'healthy living' means, Some individuals look forward to retirement as a time to 'put their feet up' and enjoy leisure time, but they may sabotage their enjoyment with lack of exercise, increasing obesity, and respiratory problems triggered by heavy smoking. Addictive gambling, over-eating, over-reliance on medication and drugs, and heavy alcohol consumption may provide an escape from loneliness and worry, Some older adults neglect themselves, are under-nourished, and experience self-inflicted neglect, perhaps because of fear, isolation, or undiagnosed mental health issues.

Active involvement (Carter and Beresford, 2010) is also seen as important for maintaining health and well-being in old age. Adult education courses, clubs for retired people, religious organisations, volunteer activities, charity work, the University of the Third Age, holidays, hobbies, sports, gardening, reading, part-time employment and family visits are examples of activities that are generally viewed as beneficial for older people's well-being.

The desire for independence: keeping control

Older people want to keep control of their lives. Older individuals whose health declines usually want to continue living in their own homes rather than move to a care home or nursing home (SCIE, 2014). Some older persons may find asking for help an almost impossible psychological task; they strive to preserve a stoic, independent attitude rather than risk feeling ashamed because they are needy and dependent (Age UK, 2017). Planning ahead is another way of keeping control.

Practice example 15.2 *A ninety-four-year-old single woman, Miss J., continued to live in the house where she had been born. Although frail, neighbours assisted her by bringing meals and helping with household tasks. Miss J. spent much of her time planning the future, organising her finances, making a will, and leaving detailed instructions designating the relatives and friends whom she wanted to receive some of her prized possessions after her death, and specifying which charities would receive donations after her death.*

Information-giving in old age

Information-giving (discussed in Chapter 7) should be an essential part of communication with older people so that they become aware of the services that are offered, the cost of the services, and which ones offer good quality. Because old age often requires planning and decision making about the future, older people need appropriate information. Their questions might include:

- Do I need help?
- What kind of help is available and where?
- How much does it cost?
- What kind of housing would meet my needs?
- Where and how can I meet people and find fulfilling activities?
- Am I eligible for grants or benefits?

Rather than present an older person with the *fait accompli of a* decision imposed on them, professional practitioners are wise to offer choice – a range of relevant information that the person can explore and use to make their own decisions.

Being alone

In old age, many people face the deaths of their husband or wife, friends, siblings, and cousins. Their parents may have died some years before. Finding oneself alone is a common dilemma of old age. Individuals live their lives as part of an age cohort or generation (e.g. 'baby boomers', 'millennials') that shares certain experiences and moments of history, but when an older age cohort begins to die, fewer people are left to share the living memories of what life was like 'in those days'. In principle, an older person can make new friends but sometimes unspoken barriers separate them from younger generations – different interests, different experiences, and different memories. Is an older person destined to live an isolated life apart from others (Davidson and Rossall, 2015)?

Practice Example 15.4 Age UK offers two types of befriending services for older people. Their service arranges for a trained volunteer to be in regular touch with an older person who lives alone. The volunteer and the older person are paired on the basis of mutual interests. The 'Call in Time' befriending is offered by telephone, and 'Face to Face' befriending involves a personal visit to the older person's home.

Difficult communication

Some older people retreat from the world, perhaps because they want to escape the legacies of their past life – broken relationships, distrust of others, fear, and anger at the world. Facing one's impending death can trigger behaviour that resembles some of Kubler-Ross' stages of loss (1969): numbness, denial, anger. Behaviour that typifies the Freudian defence mechanism of *projection* (Freud, 2018, 1936) is a frequent reaction.

Practice Example 15.3 *An older woman who had been diagnosed with incurable cancer reacted angrily to her daughter's expressions of love and offers of support, losing her temper and jeering at her daughter. Her daughter felt distraught and failed to understand why her mother was rejecting her offers of help. She did not recognise her mother's anger as a possible Freudian projection of the mother's own self-hatred onto her daughter.*

Elder abuse

Concern about child abuse in the United Kingdom escalated during the 1960s, but elder abuse – abuse in old age – was not recognised in legislation until years later. The World Health Organisation (WHO, 2018) states that about one in six people who are sixty years and older will be subject to some form of abuse in the community, and rates of elder abuse are higher in nursing homes and care homes. Elder abuse includes both physical and verbal punishment, financial fraud, or may involve giving the wrong medication, withholding medication, or restraining an older person and taking away their freedom. Action on Elder Abuse is a UK wide charity that provides general support and a national help line, assisting older people, their families, and concerned individuals to recognise the signs of abuse and how to take action.

Dementia

Dementia, one of the most difficult conditions of old age, changes the lives of individuals and their families. Rather than a single disease, dementia signifies a series of conditions that affect the functioning of the brains – progressive incurable diseases that gradually impair an individual's understanding, responsiveness, memory, and physical abilities (Andrews, 2015). Dementia's different forms include vascular dementia and Alzheimer's disease. Individuals with dementia exhibit different rates of progression and impact on their lives. Professor Tom Kitwood's Person-Centred Dementia Care (1997), developed at the University of Bradford, represented a very different approach to dementia care. Kitwood drew on Carl Rogers' person-centred therapy (1961) but applied its principles to the care of people with dementia. Person-Centred Dementia Care emphasises their personhood and individuality, and uses individualised communication to develop a relationship with the older person. Kitwood's approach is the exact opposite of a medicalised routinised approach. Person-Centred Dementia Care reminds professional practitioners that an individual with dementia is still a person.

Practice Example 15.5 *While employed at a community outreach centre in a rural Pennsylvania town, I organised a group of women to provide a social hour for long-stay patients at a state mental hospital. When we arrived at a large day ward, I observed many older women and men sitting slumped in chairs that were grouped around the walls of the ward. I was told that the patients had dementia and were unresponsive. Aware that the women who had come with me were uneasy and unsure what to do, I decided to 'model' individual contact with each of the patients. I walked up to one patient, knelt down so that I was on the same level so that she could see me clearly, and spoke to her softly. I explained who I and my colleagues were, and why we had come. Then I chatted to her on an individual basis, occasionally touching her hand. The other women who had come with me followed my example. Several of the patients gave small responses. After each of the patients had been given an opportunity for individual communication, we proceeded with the social programme.*

Feelings of loss

Feelings of loss and mourning (discussed in Chapter 12) may overwhelm some older people who are experiencing bereavement, health problems, and other crises. They may react in a stoic manner – the 'stiff upper lip' – and may offer little resistance to feelings of doom that overwhelm them. Theories that emphasise 'moving on' (Kubler-Ross, 1969) may not be as helpful as drawing on constructive theories that help to keep the lost person present in the consciousness of a bereaved person. Robert Neimeyer (2012) builds on constructive viewpoints to suggest strategies for attaining technical proficiency in grief therapy.

What do older people want from their lives?

When an older person encounters an unexpected personal crisis – a life-threatening illness, or the death of a loved one, the person may suddenly think: *what am I meant to be doing with the rest of my life?* The aftermath of a crisis leads to introspection and self-questioning. At this point, the person may become overwhelmed with sadness, or may search for a new direction for their life.

Practice Example 15.6 *An older man experienced a severe health crisis that resulted in him becoming unable to work. He began to think about the future direction of his life, and realised that he had a loving family and enough money to live on. While he was in hospital he noticed that many older patients were alone and had no visitors. He decided to become a volunteer to visit older people like those he observed in hospital.*

Some older people draw a sense of support from expressing religious beliefs that offer hope and acceptance. Their expression of spirituality sustains their searches for meaning (Mowat and O'Neill, 2013).

Different conceptual understandings of old age

Professional practitioners can benefit from increasing their awareness of different theories of ageing. Psychologists, psychiatrists, sociologists and social policy theorists offer different theories that attempt to explain the phenomenon of old age. These might be better designated as *perspectives* rather than theories because many of the concepts are insufficiently untested by research. Each perspective of ageing contributes a partial understanding rather than a comprehensive theory about growing old, and each perspective differs from each other. A brief review of some ageing theories reveals the stereotyping and negativity that have traditionally dominated perceptions of old age. Professional practitioners need to question whether their beliefs about old age signify that they have fallen into an unwitting trap of viewing older people as needy, incapable and somehow pathetic individuals.

Pessimistic and optimistic theories of old age

Some theories of old age have promoted a pessimistic view of ageing:

- Old age as a *social problem* sees ageing as both a social concern for an individual old person within society, and also a *collective* issue about the problems society faces because of the growing numbers of old people within it (MacIntyre, 1977).
- *Disengagement theory* (Cumming and Henry, 1961) suggests that ageing results in a mutual disengagement or withdrawal from contact between an older person and others, resulting in greater distance and altered relationships. Cumming and Henry imply that disengagement benefits society as a whole, because disengagement makes room for younger people to assume responsible social roles, thus freeing ageing individuals from stress. Disengagement theory has become unpopular because it apparently seems to accept and even promote the powerlessness and segregation of some older people (Estes et al, 1982).
- Age stratification (Neugarten and Neugarten, 1986) suggests that older individuals form a recognisable social group in society, and that age (Riley et al., 1972) determines social roles, power, and status.
- Socialisation (Rosow, 1974) describes a process by which individuals learn the values, customs, roles, and skills expected within their society. Ageing is seen as a time of losing established roles. Older people are assumed to reach old age with negative attitudes towards growing old that they learned as young people.
- The *political economy* of old age (Walker, 1981, Victor, 1987) argues that ageing is partly biologically determined but also socially determined by compulsory retirement and inadequate income.
- *Labelling theory* (Becker, 1963) suggests that people in society who are perceived as different are subjected to negative expectations. Older people are negatively labelled because old age is associated with unattractiveness, dependency, and death, thus triggering decreased self-esteem (Johnson, 1993, 1994).
- Ageing as a *sub-culture* (Rose, 1962) argues that older people form a distinct sub-culture within society because they interact more with each other than with other groups, experience similar problems, and are excluded from full participation in society.
- The *minority group* view of old age (Breen, 1960) argues that older people are a minority group because they experience discrimination.

More recent theories of old age adopt a more optimistic view:

- *Ageing as discovery* emerged during the late 1960s (Coleman and Bond, 1990). *Discovery* explores different experiences of old age, and emphasises that old age is non-pathological for many older people. Old age is viewed as a time for discovering new experiences, potential, and meaning. In support of the *discovery* theme, Silverman (1987) views old age as *pioneer territory*, and elderly people as *new pioneers*.
- Old age as *continuity* (Fennell, Phillipson, and Evers, 1988) recognises that the roles and issues that people experience at earlier points in their lives contribute to their ability to deal with future roles and issues; people carry forward reflections drawn from their personal histories into future events. The continuity perspective

recognises that older people's social class, gender, ethnicity, health, sexuality, religious and spiritual beliefs, and income differ.

- *Exchange* theory (Dowd, 1975) and *reciprocity* (Homans, 1974) are concerned with relationship dynamics. Dowd argues that as people become older, they lose more and more of their reciprocal power as their social roles diminish, so finally they have only the power to decide whether to comply with others' wishes.
- Activity theory (Havighurst, 1961) argues that well-being in old age depends on continuing involvement in activities. When roles are lost in old age, other activities need to be substituted to compensate for the lost roles.

The Third and Fourth Ages

The 'Third Age' describes 'the golden years' between sixty and eighty years, when individuals enjoy 'active ageing' (Lazlett, 1991) This concept is a relatively recent one, originating from a realisation that increased longevity enables more older people to remain active and find fulfilment in old age. Unlike earlier theories that emphasise poverty, loss, and illness, Lazlett's theory of old age is optimistic. He did not state a precise age when the Third and Fourth Ages begin and end, and he recognised individual differences. The Third Age is more likely to typify the life styles of older people whose income in retirement is sufficient to sustain their chosen life styles.

The 'Fourth Age' designates the years from approximately eighty years plus, when Lazlett assumed that long debilitating illnesses would reduce activity, and signal the approach of death. Yet some older people do not experience long illnesses or disability at the end of their lives, and die suddenly after a very short illness or an unexpected sudden heart attack.

Is old age a time of development?

One of the key issues of ageing is whether old age can provide opportunities for intellectual and social development. Although Freud had little to say about old age, Erikson (1950, 1986) extended the stages of development into adult life, suggesting that development continues throughout the life course. Carl Jung (1967, 1991) theorised that ongoing development in adulthood and old age is directed towards *self-actualisation* through an *individuation* process that aims to establish a *transcendent self*. Jung suggests that middle-aged people begin to re-evaluate their interests and may set new priorities, moving away from biologically determined goals of parenthood and socially determined goals of establishing themselves economically. Jung recognised gender differences in patriarchal societies, and argued that the goals of men centre on status and achievement, and women's goals centre on expressive relationships. In middle age, Jung suggests that men may become more expressive, and women may strive for worldly success. Jung emphasises reflection and introspection as personality characteristics of later life which assist in developing a *transcendent* self.

The life course: an over-arching theory

The *life course perspective* provides a framework that links separate theories together, with development exerting a reciprocal influence on a person and the environment. The life course perspective is not a theory, but presents views comprised of contributions from different disciplines. Clausen (1986) identified development, socialisation, and adaptation as three characteristics of the life course. Development is seen as multi-directional, life-long, intellectual, physical, and social. The life course incorporates concepts of social contexts, change and development in a broad vision of ageing.

Supportive services for older people: health, social care, and housing

In principle, hospitals, home-based services and GP surgeries of the National Health Service; local authority social care services, including home-based support and residential care homes; and housing services, organised by local authorities and housing associations provide a comprehensive network of services. Because health, social care, and housing are organised separately, the resulting bureaucracy, gaps in services and regional variations make it difficult for an older person to understand which services are offered in their area, which ones are free of charge, and which ones charge fees for their services. Older people know about the NHS: many of them mistakenly assume that social care services are part of the NHS and so will be provided at no cost to the individual, but social care is a means-tested service that requires most people to pay for the help they receive.

Housing services should be considered as a strategic part of health and social care. The Parliamentary Communities and Local Government Committee's report on housing for older people (CLG, 2018) called for the government to recognise the link between homes, health and social care in a forthcoming Green Paper on social care (which has been postponed several times and as of early 2019, has not been published.) The Committee urged building more housing for older people, including retirement villages, sheltered housing, and 'extra care' housing providing social care assistance and sometimes nursing care on site. Relatively few housing developments for older people in the UK offer 'through-care' or 'stepped care', enabling older individuals to live in their own small flats, and then if needed, be able to access social care services on site, and perhaps eventually move into on-site nursing care.

> Practice Example 15.6: *Lark Hill is a 'village' in Clifton, Nottingham, run by the charity Extra Care, with 327 homes for rent, purchase, or shared ownership (where a tenant has a mortgage for at least 30% of the property and pays rent for the rest). Larkhill has over 400 residents, of whom one-third have care needs, including dementia. The village provides leisure facilities as well. It received a rating of 'good' at the last Care Quality Commission inspection.*

Age-friendly communities

A World Health Organisation initiative has sought to create 'age-friendly communities' that sustain older people within their own communities. In 2006, WHO launched a global project to promote *Age-Friendly Cities*. The project identified eight domains (physical environment, housing, social environment, opportunities for participation, informal and formal community supports and health services, transportation, communication, and information) intended to establish an age-friendly community. Research by Menec et al. (2011, 2014), Liddle et al. (2014) and others explores how specific communities are developing the initiative.

Practice Example 15.7 *A United Kingdom network of Age-Friendly Communities aims to promote healthy, active ageing, and make it more possible for older individuals to remain in their own homes, keep participating in activities and contribute to their community (Centre for Ageing Better, 2019). Connecting communities who support these goals is seen as enabling more support, disseminating good practice, and sharing learning.*

Communicating with older people

This chapter has discussed prevalent attitudes towards older people, and theories that try to broaden our understanding of old age. Communicating with older people means confronting the possible barriers of one's own negative attitudes, and learning to offer respect and acceptance. This has been the major change in how old age is viewed. Gradually, a more positive acceptance of older people is beginning to emerge. The most important quality for communicating with older people is to recognise the possibility that you may hold mistaken negative assumptions about older people, and determine to overcome stereotyping them. That means being open to the recognition that older people have a right to be accepted as individuals. For example, many older people are interested in continuing sexual relationships. Some older people are gay or trans-gender.

This chapter has only touched the surface of the different aspects of ageing, and you are encouraged to continue learning about the lives and concerns of older individuals and continue exploring your attitudes. To communicate effectively with older people, a professional practitioner will:

- Avoid stereotyping an older person
- Listen carefully
- Value every older person as a distinct individual
- Encourage their discussions
- Provide appropriate information when needed
- Speak slowly and clearly and avoid rushing the older person
- Recognise older persons' reasons for rejecting offers of help
- Listen to the stories older people tell about their lives and value their communications

References

Age UK (2017) *Struggling to cope with later life Qualitative research on growing older in challenging circumstances*. BritainThinksLondon.

Age UK/NHS England (2015) *A Guide to Healthy Ageing*. https://www.england.nhs.uk/wp-content/uploads/2015/09/hlthy-ageing-brochr.pdf. Website accessed 11 February 2019.

Andrews, June (2015) *Dementia: The One-Stop Guide: Practical advice for families, professionals, and people living with dementia and Alzheimer's Disease*. Profile Books: London.

Becker, H. (1963) *Outsiders: Studies in the Sociology of Deviance*. Free Press: New York.

Breen, L. Z. (1960) 'The Aging Individual' in Tibbitts, C.T. (ed.), *Handbook of Social Gerontology*. University of Chicago Press: Chicago, pp. 1–17.

Carter, T. and Beresford, P. (2010) *Age and Change: Models of involvement for older people*. Joseph Rowntree Foundation: York.

Centre for Ageing Better (2019) *UK Network of Age-Friendly Communities.* https://www.ageing-better.org.uk/age-friendly-communities, website accessed 10 February 2019.

Clausen, J. (1986) *The Life Course: A Sociological Perspective.* Pearson: London.

CLG Communities and Local Government Committee (2018) *Housing for older people Second Report.* House of Commons: London.

Coleman, Peter and Bond, John (eds) (1990) *Ageing in Society: An introduction to Social Gerontology.* Sage: London.

Collins, Patricia Hill, and Bilge, Sirma (2016) *Intersectionality.* Polity Press: Cambridge.

Cumming, E. and Henry, W.E. (1961) Growing *Old: The Process of Disengagement.* Basic Books: New York.

Davidson, Susan and Rossall, Phil (2015) *Evidence Review: Loneliness in Later Life.* Age UK: London.

Dowd, J.P. (1975) 'Ageing as Exchange: A Preface to Theory', *Journal of Gerontology,* Volume 80, Issue 4, pp. 584–594.

Erikson, E. (1950, 1986) *Childhood and Society.* Norton: New York.

Estes, C.Swan, J. and Gerard, L. (1982). 'Dominant and competing paradigms in gerontology: Towards a political economy of ageing', *Ageing and Society,* Volume 12, pp. 151–164.

Fennell, G., Phillipson, C. and Evers, H. (1988) *The Sociology of Old Age.* Open University Press: Milton Keynes.

Freud, A. (2018, 1936) *The Ego and the Mechanisms of Defense.* Abingdon: Routledge.

Freud, S. (1986) *The Essentials of Psycho-analysis, selected by Anna Freud.* Penguin: London.

Havighurst, R. J. (1961) 'Successful ageing', *The Gerontologist,* Volume 1, pp. 8–13.

HM Government (2010) *Healthy Lives Healthy People: Our Strategy for Public Health in England*>https://assets.publishing.service.gov.uk/government/uploads/system/uploads/attachment_data/file/216096/dh_127424.pdf

Homans, G. (1974) *Social Behaviour,* 2nd Edition. Harcourt Brace Jovanovich: New York.

Johnson, M. (1993) 'Dependency and interdependency' in Bond, J., Coleman, P. and Peace, S. (eds), *Ageing in Society.* Sage Publications: London, pp. 255–279.

Johnson, M. L. (1995). 'Interdependency and the generational compact', *Ageing and Society,* Volume 15, Issue 2, pp. 243–265. Jung, C. G. (1967). *The Development of Personality.* Collected Works. Volume 17. 1991 Edition. Routledge: London.

Kitwood, Tom (1997) *Dementia Reconsidered: The Person Comes First.* Open University Press: London.

Kubler-Ross, E. (1969) *On Death and Dying.* Macmillan: New York.

Laslett, P. (1991) *A fresh map of life: The emergence of the third age.* Harvard University Press: Cambridge, MA.

Liddle, Jennifer, Scharf, Thomas, Bartlam, Bernadette, Bernard, Miriam, and Sim, Julius (2014) 'Exploring the Friendliness of Purpose-Built Retirement Communities: Evidence from England', *Ageing & Society,* Volume 34, Issue 9,October 2014, pp. 1601–1629.

MacIntyre, S. (1977) 'Old age as a social problem' in Dingwall, R., Heath, C., Reid, M., and Stacey, M. (eds), *Health Care and Health Knowledge.* Croom Helm: London.

Menec, Verena H., Hutton, Louise, Newall, Nancy, Nowicki, Scott John, and Veselyuk, Dawn (2014) 'How "age-friendly" are rural communities and what community characteristics are related to age-friendliness? The case of rural Manitoba Canada', *Ageing & Society,* Volume 34, Part 9, September.

Menec, Verena H., Means, Robin, Keating, Norah, Parkhurst, Graham, and Eales, Jacquie (2011) 'Conceptualising Age-Friendly Communities', *Canadian Journal on Aging,* Volume 30, Issue 3, September 2011, pp. 479–493.

Mowat, Harriet, and O'Neill, Maureen (2013) *Spirituality and ageing: Implications for the care and support of older people.* Insight 19, IRISS: Glasgow.

Neimeyer, Robert (2012) 'Presence, Process, and Procedure. A Relational Frame for Technical Proficiency in Grief Therapy', in Neimeyer, Robert (ed.), *Techniques of Grief Therapy.* Routledge: New York, pp. 3–11.

Neugarten, B. L. and Neugarten, D. A. (1986). 'Age in the aging society'. Daedalus, Volume 115, Issue1, pp. 31–49.

Phillips, J., Ajrouch, K. and Hillcoat-Nalletanby, S. (2010) *Key Concepts in Social Gerontology*. Sage: London.

RileyM. W., JohnsonM., FonerA. (1972) 'A sociology of age stratification', *Aging and society*, Volume 3. Russell Sage Foundation: New York.

Rogers, Carl (1961) *On Becoming a Person*. Constable: London.

Rose, A.M. (1962) 'The subculture of the aging, a topic for sociological research', *Gerontologist*, Volume 2, pp. 123–127.

Rosow, Irving (1974) *Socialization to Old Age*. University of California Press: Berkeley.

SCIE Social Care Institute for Excellence (2014) *Commissioning home care for older people*. Guide 54. SCIE: London.

Silverman, Philip (1987) 'Introduction: The Life Course Responsibility', in *The Elderly as Modern Pioneers*. Indiana University Press: Bloomington, Indiana.

The Pensions Advisory Service (2019) *The State Pension: Know your State Pension Age*https://www.pensionsadvisoryservice.org.uk/about-pensions/the-state-pension/know-your-state-pension-age. Website accessed 10 February 2019.

Townsend, Peter (1958) 'A society for people' in N. MacKenzie (ed.), *Conviction*. MacGibbon and Kee: London.

Victor, Christina (1987) *Old age in modern society: a textbook of social gerontology*. Croom Helm: London.

Walker, Alan (1981) 'Towards a Political Economy of Old Age', *Ageing and Society*, Volume 1, Issue 1, pp. 73–94.

WHO World Health Organisation (2018) *Elder Abuse*https://www.who.int/en/news-room/fact-sheets/detail/elder-abuse. Website accessed 12 December 2019.

WHO, US National Institute of Aging (2011) *Global Health and Ageing*. https://www.who.int/ageing/publications/global_health.pdf. Website accessed 11 February 2019.

World Health Organisation (2014) *Active Ageing: a Policy Framework*. Website accessed 10 February 2019.https://extranet.who.int/agefriendlyworld/wp-content/uploads/2014/06/WHO-Active-Ageing-Framework.pdf

Communicating with individuals with mental health issues, physical impairments or learning difficulties

The long history of neglect and institutionalisation

Achieving effective, ethical communication means learning about the long history of neglect (Means and Smith, 1994) that characterised health and social care provision for people with physical impairments, learning difficulties, or mental health issues. The chapter begins by reviewing the history of service provision. 'Disability' and 'mental illness' were conditions that were feared in the ancient and medieval world. People believed that these individuals were possessed by the devil or were 'witches'. Some of these attitudes linger on in our contemporary evidence-based society.

> Practice Example 16.1: *A fifteen-year-old girl who lived in a children's home told a visitor to the home about her diagnosis of Huntingdon's Chorea, an inherited progressive disease that usually reveals itself during childhood or adulthood and results in an early death. Her mother had died of the disease, and her father had died of a heart attack. The girl seemed matter of fact, but subdued, explaining that this was why she was living in the children's home. She showed little emotion. The visitor inwardly felt afraid and horrified when she heard the girl's story, and found it difficult to maintain a conversation with her.*
>
> Question: *What might have been an appropriate response to the girl's revelation?*

In the nineteenth and twentieth centuries, long stay institutions provided flawed 'solutions' for the perceived 'problems' of 'the mentally ill', 'the disabled' and 'the mentally handicapped'. (The traditional language to designate these individuals is notable for its denial of their personhood). Means and Smith (1994, pp. 17–18) called these the 'Cinderella services' that waited in vain for a fairy godmother to transform them. The workhouse of the nineteenth century was an institution for the destitute, intended to deter individuals (labelled 'paupers') from failing to work. Their destitution and poverty were attributed to moral failure, not adverse economic and social conditions or disability. Individuals were blamed for their own poverty. People with physical impairments, learning difficulties, or mental health issues because of advanced age, accidents, illness, or disablement from birth also risked being sent to the workhouse – like a punishment for their existence.

Attitudes began to change slowly when society acknowledged that many destitute inmates of the workhouse were people who were unable to work or who had been forced out of employment by economic circumstances. Within some workhouses, attempts were made to provide more specialist provision for older people, people with a physical impairment, learning difficulties, mental health issues, and children. Some workhouses eventually became public assistance hospitals. However, families of destitute workhouse inmates or long stay hospital patients, as well as relatives of destitute individuals in the community, were expected to maintain them financially. Gradually old-age pensions were introduced, giving older people a means of support.

During the First World War, the disabling injuries and 'shell shock' of many returning servicemen exposed the lack of resources for their care. During the Second World War, the inadequacies of health and social care provision were exacerbated by widespread destruction and loss of lives that left many people homeless (Kesternich et al., 2014).

After the end of the Second World War in 1945, introduction of a National Health Service and a National Assistance Act led to the transfer of workhouse inmates to long stay hospitals and residential care homes run by health and welfare committees. Families were no longer made responsible for patients' and residents' financial support. Many former workhouse buildings, although inadequate, became long stay hospitals or residential homes, and these buildings were used for many decades.

> Practice Example 16.2 *My first placement as a postgraduate social work student was in a hospital that had been a workhouse and which still retained many institutional features. Later, in my first social work role, I visited long stay mental health patients in large institutions that had been part of the old public assistance and workhouse system. Locked wards in mental hospitals and hospitals for people with learning disabilities were common features. Many of the patients were elderly, single women, and I was told that some had been institutionalised in their youth because they had become pregnant whilst unmarried.*

Changing attitudes

Attitudes began to change. Research publications exposed the neglect and harshness of institutions – Peter Townsend's *The Last Refuge* (1962), Erving Goffman's *Asylums* (1961), and Pauline Morris' *Put Away* (1969) were some of these publications. Their books became widely read, and created growing public concern about inadequate institutional standards. As Means and Smith (1994) point out, the reforms brought about by the Children Act 1948 can be contrasted with reluctance to create similar changes for adults with physical impairments, learning difficulties, or mental health issues.

> Practice Example 16.3 *My beginning a career as a social worker illustrates the unequal resources provided for adults, compared to children. After making several applications for my first job as a qualified social worker, I was offered a post in a Children's Department with children, young people and their families, and a post in a Public Health Department with adults who were impaired by physical conditions, age, or by learning difficulties. The post in the Children's Department paid more, offered regular supervision, smaller case loads, and employed qualified social workers. In contrast, the Public Health Department post was not as well paid, had higher case loads, employed relatively few qualified social workers, and supervision was not a highlighted feature. The choice was obvious: I*

accepted the post in the Children's Department, and worked there for four years, observing the continuing but gradually eroding existence of institutionalisation, and feeling that I was part of a reforming movement that would improve standards.

Moving away from institutionalisation

Care in the community began to become a reality in the late 1960s and 1970s, but progress in replacing institutional care was slow. Progress was assisted by advances in bio-medical sciences that resulted in anti-psychotic medication, anti-depressant drugs and tranquillisers becoming available to treat mental health conditions. The sight of patients being kept in restraining straightjackets because they might cause harm to themselves or to others used to be a frequent occurrence before these medications became available.

Practice Example 16.4 After working for the Children's Department in England, I moved to the USA. I applied for social work posts there, and one job that was offered was with a large state hospital for 'the handicapped and mentally ill' which now wanted to resettle its patients in the community. I toured some of the wards before my formal interview, and observed large wards with individuals of all ages, many of whom had lived in the hospital since infancy. I saw individuals with hydrocephaly, conjoined twins, disfiguring physical conditions, Down's syndrome, and a range of other conditions. Their world – the only world they knew – was the hospital. What was needed to help them live happily in the community and realise the goal of community care? I was not given much assurance of a clear strategy for achieving this. I did not accept this post, and instead was employed in a community-based role running a multi-service outreach centre that tried to respond positively to drug and alcohol addiction, mental health issues, and people with physical impairments and learning difficulties that lived in the community.

The new Social Services Departments that were established in 1971 to unite local authorities' children's and adults' services continued the predominance of children's services, in part because of growing concerns about child protection and safeguarding. (Adult safeguarding legislation, in contrast, was not passed until several years after children's safeguarding laws.) The Community Care Act 1990 supported a policy shift towards providing home-based services and community-based services in small units, rather than in large institutions, but lack of resources to meet growing demands because of population growth and people's increasing longevity hindered achievement of the Act's aims. The plight of single older women was worse than that of older men because of their lower incomes. The Act operated in tandem with the National Assistance Act 1948, the Chronically Sick and Disabled Person's Act 1970, the Community Care (Direct Payments) Act 1996, and the Community Care (Delayed Discharges) Act 2003. This incremental growth of provision led to complexities and anomalies of implementation.

The Community Care Act (2014) requires local authorities to ensure that adults are able to obtain services that prevent their needs from becoming more serious, receive appropriate information and advice to enable them to make appropriate decisions for their care, and can choose from a range of services. The 2014 Act gives local authorities a co-ordinating role that requires them to become aware of the range of services (health services, charities, voluntary services) in their areas, rather than focus only on their directly provided services. The problem is that spending on health and social care services has not kept pace with the rising demand and the new legislative ambitions. Arguably, resources for adult services continue to lag behind, and this is especially evident in the difficulties of recruiting sufficient numbers of social care workers for adult hostels, residential homes, and home-based care services (Moriarty et al., 2018).

Both in the UK and the USA, community groups and voluntary agencies have been established to express the needs and wishes of individuals who had been subject to institutional power and not fully recognised as human beings. The voices of 'experts by experience' – service users and patients – have begun to make a difference. Change is still needed. The *Guardian* (Salman, 2019) reported that some people with learning difficulties and autism still live in locked units that are meant to provide therapeutic care and support to those who have moved from long-term institutional care. *Rightful Lives*, a human rights campaign, claims that local authorities and NHS clinical commissioning groups continue to use these secure units instead of finding appropriate support in the community.

Communicating with individuals who have mental health issues

Mental health issues range from mild depression and anxiety to severe depressive symptoms, eating disorders, and to psychotic illnesses, where the individual's thought patterns and behaviour become disorganised and irrational. Society's understanding of mental illness is changing, and it can be argued that definitions of mental illness are to some extent, socially constructed. The question is: how does a society define – and who in that society has the right to define – what is 'normal' or 'abnormal' behaviour, and if judged 'abnormal', what kind of care and treatment should be offered? Thomas Szasz (1920–2012), a Hungarian-American psychiatrist, wrote passionately against what he described as the coercion and over-medicalisation of mental health patients (1961), gaining a reputation of being 'anti-psychiatry' but also prompting the rise of patient advocates to support mental health patients, and triggering challenges to the power of the medical establishment. Szasz argued that illness applied only to the body, not the mind, but he was in favour of voluntary psychotherapy as a healing strategy.

Practice Example 11.2 *Whilst working as the manager of a community-based mental health outreach centre in a small town in Pennsylvania, I attended regular staff development seminars at the Reading (PA) Hospital Mental Health Treatment Center. During one seminar, I listened to Dr. Szasz, who was the guest speaker. He spoke passionately about his 'anti-psychiatry' views, and also about the 'disease model' of homosexuality, which he opposed (homosexuality was, at that time, classified as a mental illness). A few months later, Dr. Rotenberg, the hospital psychiatrist who had invited Thomas Szasz, announced that the American Psychiatric Association had decided, by a majority vote, that homosexuality was no longer a mental illness. His bemused tone suggested to me that he recognised the point of Szasz' arguments – after all, if the 'mental illness' of homosexuality could be voted out by a majority of physicians, did that mean that other categories of mental illness could also be voted out because a majority of doctors thought that certain symptoms and behaviours were no longer to be considered a mental illness?*

The social context of this event is to understand the role that the DSM (Diagnostic and Statistical Manual of Mental Disorders) plays in determining the power and scope of USA medical care. (Note that the United Kingdom does not use the DSM, but classifies illnesses according to the ICD – International Classification of Diseases, published by the World Health Organisation – a manual used in many countries world-wide.) Established in 1952, the DSM (now in its fifth edition) sets out the classification of mental disorders, using standard criteria and language. Over the years, the number of illnesses categorised in the DSM has expanded, and more and more conditions have become diagnosable 'mental illnesses', resulting in the growth and influence of international pharmaceutical firms. The DSM has been criticised for over-medicalising human conditions, but their inclusion in the DSM means that American citizens with these conditions will be able to obtain funding for treatment (important in a country lacking a national health service). In the present day, recognised categories of mental illness include anxiety disorders (phobias and obsessive-compulsive disorders), mood disorders (depression and anxiety), personality disorders (paranoid, narcissistic, anti-social), dis-associative disorders (amnesia, multiple personality), psychotic disorders (schizophrenia), and organic brain disorders (diseases, brain injury).

More in the spirit of Thomas Szasz, in 2018 the Division of Clinical Psychology of the British Psychological Society published *The Power Threat Meaning Framework* written by psychologists Lucy Johnstone and Mary Boyle, who intend the Framework to represent a paradigm shift away from the current classification systems of the DSM and ICD, which they regard as flawed. The Framework provides a conceptual alternative to medicalised assumptions, focussing instead on the underlying meanings of lived experiences, and the relationships between individual distress and wider social and cultural contexts. Significantly, the project team included 'survivor' and carer perspectives, as well as professional practitioners and researchers. The aim of the Framework is to support the construction of non-diagnostic, non-blaming stories about strength and survival and 'to re-integrate many behaviours and reactions currently diagnosed as symptoms of mental disorder back into the range of universal human experience' (Johnstone and Boyle, 2018, p. 5).

People with mental health problems were, in the past (and sometimes are today), feared and misunderstood. In previous centuries, people with mental illnesses were sent to an asylum or a mental hospital to live in locked wards away from the general population. The stigma associated with mental illness meant that many individuals hid their symptoms and feared being ostracised or taken away against their will if they openly sought help. A generation ago, after the development of modern anti-psychotic drugs and tranquillizers that helped to abate some of the severe symptoms of mental illness, and with the publication of mental health research (Goffman, 1961) that exposed the institutionalisation of individuals in mental health hospitals, new legislation began to change how people with mental illnesses were treated. Hospitals started to empty out, and some mental health institutions closed altogether.

Now many more people with mental illnesses are able to live in the community on their own or in group homes with some supervision. People with mental health issues are free individuals. Some individuals may decide that they do not want to continue taking their medication, may refuse treatment, and may want to move away from their sheltered living environment. Some of these individuals may eventually become homeless. Recognising how human individuality and a person's personal and social contexts influence their personal decisions is relevant to understanding these situations.

Although society acknowledges the issues of providing sufficient appropriate help and support to people with unrecognised and untreated mental illness, it struggles to meet increasing demands for support. Currently concerns have been expressed about the numbers of people in the population who have a mental health problem. NHS Digital (2014) estimates that one-sixth of the population in England (aged 16–64 years) has a mental health problem. The report states that mental health problems are increasing, that the problems begin early in life, and that the incidence of more severe types of mental illness has risen in the last twenty years. Women are more likely to be affected, and young people are said to be particularly vulnerable. Men are more likely to commit suicide. The report argues that mental health services are under-funded in comparison to other areas of health.

When a person needs urgent mental health treatment and is judged to be at risk of harm to themselves and/or to others, he or she can be detained ('sectioned') for treatment without their consent under the Mental Health Act (1983). In December 2018, Parliament announced plans to revise the Mental Health Act, so that the legislation includes provisions that would enable individuals to agree statutory Advance Choice Documents in which they state their preferences for any future in-patient care, and are able to challenge their treatment at a legally aided tribunal. The future reforms are intended to give the patient more voice and enable the patient's views to carry more weight (BASW, 2018).

Professional practitioners in a range of roles are likely to encounter individuals with mental health issues, not all of whom have been diagnosed or offered treatment. Social workers and some health practitioners may practise as Approved Mental Health Professionals (AMHP) who are specially trained to assess and make recommendations about compulsory detention. Counsellors may work for the NHS to deliver the IAPT programme – Improved Access to Psychological Therapies.

It is crucial to build individual and public tolerance towards people with a mental illness and not fear them or demonise them as they have often been in the past. Every practitioner needs to learn more about how to communicate effectively with these individuals. The principles of good communication apply to people with mental health issues, but practitioners need to be aware that people whose illness impairs their logical thinking may not always respond well to Rogers' person-centred approach. Their thinking may be scattered, impaired, and suspicious. They may deny their mental illnesses, but that is not a reason to abandon them entirely.

Practitioners should become familiar with the characteristics of mental illnesses, which too frequently are undiagnosed and untreated. Realistic goals include building trust, working in partnership with other professions, and supporting and sustaining individuals with mental health problems to obtain appropriate help and support. Communication needs to be non-stigmatising and respectful of the humanity of the person. Fear of violence and threatening behaviour is a realistic emotion amongst those who try to help others, and practitioner knowledge should include strategies to keep themselves and others safe.

Autism and Asperger's syndrome

Some mental health conditions are relatively newly identified. Autism is a mental health condition that was first described in 1943 and 1944. Autism is a range or spectrum of behaviours that differ in characteristics and severity from one individual to another. Autistic people characteristically have difficulties with social communication and inter-action, and can exhibit repetitive behaviour.

Steve Silberman's prize-winning book, *Neurotribes: The legacy of autism and how to think smarter about people who think differently* (2015), which won the Samuel Johnson Prize, tells the story of autism and Asperger's syndrome. Silberman, an American journalist, listened and talked to parents, children, physicians, teachers, and autistic people themselves, many of whom are living successful lives, and learned about their support systems. His book pays tribute to the efforts of parents that helped to improve public and professional atti-tudes and gained more support for individuals with autism.

Two Austrian-born doctors separately identified the condition during the Second World War, one in the USA, the other in Vienna. In 1943, Dr. Leo Kanner, a con-sultant paediatric psychiatrist at Johns Hopkins Hospital in Baltimore, Maryland, pub-lished a paper about children who exhibited repetitious obsessive behaviours and who preferred to be alone. He called the children's condition *early infantile autism*, or *autism,* as it is now widely known. In 1944 in Austria, Dr. Hans Asperger, a Viennese paediatrician, published a paper about a syndrome characterised by repetitive behaviours and difficulties in social communication. This became known eventually as Asperger's syndrome, but the syndrome was not widely acknowledged until after the end of the Second World War, because Asperger's initial paper was published in German. After Asperger's research was translated into English and other languages, Asperger's syndrome became recognised worldwide in 1981.

Silberman's book is partly a detective story about the origins of this condition, and a critique of some early theories about its cause. Kanner had initially believed that the con-dition was triggered by a mother's cold behaviour – the 'refrigerator mother' theory, which is now discredited. This theory was popularised by Bruno Bettelheim, a Viennese-born psychiatrist who had been imprisoned in German concentration camps before emi-grating to the USA in 1939. Bettleheim expanded on Kanner's 'refrigerator mother' in his book *The Empty Fortress* (1967) in which he attributed the cause of autism to lack of par-ental love and attention to the child. Bettelheim was popular and well known in the USA for his therapeutic work with children, but after he died in 1990, he was accused of pla-giarism, false academic qualifications, and abusive treatments of his patients.

Silberman argues that Bettleheim's espousal of this cause did not help autistic people and their parents. The second part of Silberman's book tells how the parents of autistic children in the USA have helped to change perceptions of this condition, dispelled some of the early negative beliefs, have won recognition of the talents of autistic individuals (many of whom now work in the computer industry), and promoted their acceptance. Understanding and treatment of the condition – or range of conditions – have expanded over the years and are widely recognised today. Our knowledge of autism has grown and is growing.

Listening to the voices of mental health survivors

Two recent books, written by survivors of long-term anxiety and depression, portray their struggles to carry on, and their searches for meaning. Scott Stossel, editor of the *Atlantic* magazine in New York, wrote *My Age of Anxiety: Fear, hope, dread, and the search for peace of mind* (2013) which became a best-seller in the USA. He tells the story of his life-long struggle with acute anxiety and the help he sought, but more than that, he explores with honesty and in great depth his family history, how anxiety affects certain individuals, including himself, and discusses historic persons who experienced anxiety and what they did about it. He recounts his search for help and his experience with the many different medications and types of therapy he tried over the years. Nothing, it seems, succeeded in fully abating his anxiety. Yet, throughout this time he was successful in his career and was happily married. The book concludes not with a magic cure but with Scott's current therapist commenting that Scott has resilience, and Scott recognising that he has been able to live with his anxiety. He tells the reader that although his wife wishes he wasn't so anxious, she worries that he might become a 'jerk' if he lost his anxiety – his anxiety has somehow enabled him to be more sensitive towards others.

Johann Hari, a British journalist, wrote *Lost Connections: Uncovering the real causes of depression – and the unexpected solutions* (2018). He tells the story of the depression he experienced from childhood. He took prescribed medication for his depression for many years and saw a therapist, but despite the medication, his depression continued. The book portrays his odyssey of discovery – his search for meaning and understanding of his depression. He began to ask himself whether depression is caused by a chemical imbalance in the brain, as he had always believed, or whether there are other contributory factors. His book discusses his travels and conversations with many different people all over the world who helped him to expand his understanding of depression. Hari identifies nine causal factors for the disconnection of people from each other, which exacerbate the individual risks of becoming depressed or anxious. The nine factors centre on *disconnection*: from meaningful work; from other people; from meaningful values; from childhood trauma; from status and respect; from the natural world; from a hopeful or secure future; from the real role of genes; and from the real role of brain changes. Hari does not reject the use of medication, but he developed his understanding of the importance of human interconnection and the search for meaning as strategies for combating depression.

Physical impairment: the increasing power of service users

Some individuals with physical impairments became writers and academics whose publications helped to change negative attitudes. Michael Oliver, Tom Shakespeare (2014), Vic Finkelstein (2001) and others conceptualised issues in ways that had significant meaning to people with a disability. Their efforts helped to strengthen service user movements for physical disabilities, learning disabilities and mental health issues. Over time, service users' influence on service provision grew as they became active members of service user groups, health services' governing bodies, social work course committees, and other organisational bodies. (Although service user representation is well established in the Health Service and in social services departments, counselling organisations currently lack significant service user representation.)

Practice Example 16.5 *Shaping Our Lives National User Network is an example of a user organisation that enables the voices of users of services to be heard. The Network works with people with physical and/or sensory impairments, learning difficulties, users and survivors of mental, users and survivors of mental health services, young people with experience of being 'looked after', people living with HIV/AIDS or life limiting illnesses, older people, people with experience of alcohol and drug services, and homeless people (Shaping Our Lives Website, 2019).*

Professor Peter Beresford, Co-Chair of Shaping Our Lives, has expressed concern about the closure of user-led organisations, and warns that they are facing a threat of extinction because they are being side-lined from government consultations and funded projects. More than 150 member groups have been lost in the last two years, according to the National Survivor User Network (NSUN). Beresford argues that austerity cuts, a government shift towards privatisation and the dominance of a few large charities that are run like big businesses makes it more difficult for small, local, accountable user-led organisations and disabled people's user-led organisations to survive. He called for a radical review of both government and funding policies (Pring, 2019, *Disability News Service Website*. Accessed 19 March 2019).

Learning how to communicate effectively: the importance of language

As well as learning about the history of service provision and the predominant attitudes, effective communication depends on being able to choose suitable language for interactions with others. Michael Oliver (1945–2019), who was Professor Emeritus of Disability Studies at the University of Greenwich, drew attention to issues about the language that society uses to define 'disabled people'. He acknowledged (1996, p. 5) that what is 'acceptable language' can change over time. (Although I have tried to choose my words carefully when writing the chapters of this book, I realised that I might not have always succeed in selecting acceptable contemporary language, and I apologise for any unintended inaccuracies.)

> Practice Example 16.6 In 1952, parents of children with cerebral palsy founded the Spastics Society (with the help of social workers) to improve their children's opportunities for education and care. In an example of growing sensitivity to the use of descriptive language, in 1994 the Society changed its name to Scope, a less stigmatising designation, after a two-year consultation with service users and trustees. Scope's purpose broadened to include supporting the social model of disability, campaigning and challenging negative attitudes to disability, as well as providing direct services (Scope, 2019. Websitehttps://www.scope,org.uk,accessed 17 March 2019).

Oliver supported the Union of Physically Impaired Against Segregation's (UPIAS) distinction between *impairment* and *disability*, that *impairment* is 'lacking part of or all of a limb, or having a defective limb, organism or mechanism of the body' and *disability* is 'the disadvantage or restriction of activity caused by contemporary organisations which take no or little account of people who have physical impairments and thus excludes them from the mainstream of social activities'. Oliver defined 'disabled people' (1996, p. 5) as having three elements: the presence of impairment, the experience of restrictions that are externally imposed, and self-identification as a disabled person.

Oliver also developed a key concept that he derived from the UPIAS definitions of disability and impairment – the *social model*, which locates the causes of disability within society; and its opposite, the *individual* or *medical* model (1996, pp. 30–42) that attributes problems to the functional limitations of disabilities. The *social model* helped to change society's thinking about disability. Oliver later questioned whether the social model was becoming a strait jacket, responding to criticisms that the model cannot always connect with the actual experience of impairment, and its denial of the pain of impairment and failure to include the oppressions of racism, sexism, and homophobia (pp. 37–39). Oliver accepted that the social model cannot 'do everything' (p. 41). Social work practitioners too often interpret the *social model* and the *medical model* with an overly simplistic meaning that separates it from disability, with the *social model* portrayed as representing social work's tolerant, accepting approach, in contrast to the *medical model* which is portrayed as the supposedly rigid aspects of health care. Little awareness is demonstrated of the changes in the Health Service which promote community-based services and patient representation. This interpretation of the social model reinforces oppositional thinking rather than collaboration between health and social care.

The practice of communication

How should a professional practitioner communicate with an individual with a physical impairment, a learning difficulty, or a mental health issue? The first step is to confront your own private beliefs and assumptions about these individuals and begin to acquire new knowledge about the impact of historic institutionalisation and neglect on their lives, so that you perceive them as human beings with human needs. The early part of this chapter may help to fill in some gaps, but it is hoped that you will further explore their history and their present conditions. Once you become aware of our shared humanity, you can begin by seeking to create an honest supportive relationship between you and an individual with a physical impairment, a learning difficulty, or a mental illness. The relationship will require awareness, sensitivity, sharing of knowledge, and collaboration.

> *Practice Example 16.7 An eighty-three-year-old widow, who had become physically impaired through a stroke but who retained her intellectual abilities, decided to move to a nursing home. Her three adult children went with her to visit a number of different establishments. At one nursing home, whose interior was new, shiny and bright, a senior nurse with a clipboard ushered the widow and her family into an interview room. The nurse began asking questions rapidly about the widow's health and abilities, but did not address the widow directly, instead directing her questions to the widow's adult children. 'Is she incontinent?' 'Does she wander at night?' After ten minutes, the widow's son stood up and said: 'We're leaving. You have not once looked at my mother, or called her by her name, and you have asked many questions about her daily habits as if she is not in the room. This tells me that my mother would not receive good care in this establishment, because you do not acknowledge her as a human being.'*

This is an almost classic example of professional communication gone wrong, and sadly, it is a true example of quite recent practice. Examples of this kind of practice have been written about for years (e.g. *does he take sugar?*) to illuminate the pitfalls of failing to recognise that persons with an impairment, a learning difficulty, or a mental health issue are human beings and must be recognised as such.

The list of 'dos and don'ts' for establishing good communication is potentially endless, because the individuality of each person and situation will differ. The following pointers comprise only a very small sample of how to communicate in a professional and ethical manner. Good communication requires a professional practitioner to

- respect the person's humanity.
- introduce yourself clearly and slowly, explain your role and the purpose of the meeting, and how the meeting will proceed.
- note the two-way communication between the person and yourself, including the person's non-verbal expressions of doubt or anxiety, verbal flatness or anger. Seek to address these indicative feelings in a non-judgemental, non-confrontational manner. Remember that many individuals fear being blamed and becoming the target of disapproval.
- If you are communicating with a person who is deaf and can lip-read, speak slowly, with your face and lips well illuminated. Sit so that the person can see you clearly; or if the person cannot lip read but has some hearing, ask how they want you to communicate. Use speech that is clear and not too fast, and/or write notes for the person to read. Take as much time as is needed, and don't rush.
- If you are communicating with a person who has little or no vision, introduce yourself, and preview your physical movements as you go along. Avoid touching the person without warning or permission. Do not rush to offer physical assistance unless you ask first if that is what the person wants.
- Do not stand or sit at a height above someone in a wheel chair.
- Do not shout as if the person is not able to understand you. Speak slowly and clearly.
- Avoid using professional jargon. The person may not wish to admit that they are not able to understand complex explanations stated in technical language, and spoken very fast.
- Explain according to the person's ability to understand – but you will need to determine after you get to know the person whether you need to explain some information in simple language. Don't assume beforehand.
- Allow time for questions.
- Try to voice their possible fears as a way of ascertaining their feelings and check whether your hunch is correct.
- Remember that some impairments may be invisible at first sight – dyslexia, and autism for example.
- Don't assume a 'pecking order' of valuing certain conditions above others, or devaluing or doubting the verity of a person's condition – for example, mental health issues like anxiety and depression can easily be wrongly attributed to moral and character failings.
- Learn how to protect your own safety and that of the person, if a situation becomes emotionally overwrought.

Summarising the chapter

This chapter has provided an overview of traditional punitive and fearful attitudes towards individuals with a physical impairment, a learning difficulty or a mental health issue. The chapter argues that they are, above all, human beings with human rights, and that provides the key to good communication. Professional practitioners must recognise their intrinsic worth. The availability of anti-psychotic drugs to abate the symptoms of severe mental illnesses made it possible to close large long stay hospitals that had shut these individuals away from the rest of the world. The voices of people with impairments, learning difficulties, and mental health issues began to be heard from within user-led organisations. Their support of *the social model of disability* helped to dispel negative images of their identities and has ended their exclusion from society.

Effective communication is built on sharing knowledge, being aware of the person's feelings, being sensitive to their hopes and fears, and collaborating with them on shared goals. Communication means listening to the views of service users, responding to them with acceptance, and working with them to help bring about further positive changes.

References

Asperger, Hans (1944). 'Die Autistisehen Psychopathen im Kindesalter', *Arch. Psych. Nervenkrankh*, Volume 117, pp. 76–136.

Beresford, P. (2016) *All Our Welfare: Towards Participatory Social Policy*. Policy Press: London.

Beresford, Peter (2019) 'User-led sector faces threat of extinction', *Disability News Service. Accessed* 28 January 2018, https://www.disabilitynewsservice.com/user-led-sector-faces-threat-of-extinction/

Bettleheim, Bruno (1967) *The Empty Fortress: Infantile Autism and the Birth of the Self: Infantile Autism and the Birth of Self*. The Free Press (Simon and Schuster): New York.

BASW British Association of Social Workers (2018) 'Reform Mental Health Act to give more power to patients'. *Professional Social Work*. BASW: Birmingham. December 2018/January 2019, p. 7.

Finkelstein, V. (2001) 'A Personal Journey Into Disability Politics'. Leeds University Centre for Disability Studies: Leeds. Accessed 26 January 2018, http://www.independentliving.org/docs3/finkelstein01a.pdf

Goffman, E. (1961) *Asylums: Essays on the Condition of the Social Situation of Mental Patients and Other Inmates*. Anchor Books: New York.

Hari, Johann (2018) *Lost Connections. Uncovering the real causes of depression – and the unexpected solutions*. Bloomsbury Publishing: London.

Johnstone, Lucy and Boyle, Mary (2018) *The Power Threat Meaning Framework Division of Clinical Psychology*. The British Psychological Society: Leicester.

Kanner, L. (1943) 'Affective disturbances of affective contact', *The Nervous Child*, Volume 2, pp. 217–250.

Kesternich, I., Siflinger, B., Smith, J.P., and Winter, J.K. (2014) 'The Effects of World War II on Economic and Health Outcomes across Europe', *Review of Economics and Statistics*1 March, Volume 96, Issue 1, pp. 103–118.

Kropowska, Juliet (2010) *Communication and Interpersonal Skills in Social Work* (Transforming Social Work Practice Series). Learning Matters/Sage: London.

McCorry, L. and Mason, J. (2011) *Communication Skills for the Healthcare Professional*. Lipppincott Williams & Wilkins: Philadelphia.

Means, Robin and Smith, Randall (1994) *Community Care. Policy and Practice*. Macmillan: Basingstoke and London.

Means, Robin, Richards, Sally, and Smith, Randall (2008) *Community Care. Policy and Practice*. Palgrave Macmillan: London.

Moriarty, Jo, Manthorpe, Jill, and Harris, Jess (2018) *Recruitment and retention in adult social care services*. King's College Policy Institute. Social Care Workforce Unit: London.

Morris, Pauline (1969) *Put Away: Institutions for the Mentally Retarded*. Routledge Kegan Paul: London.

Moss, Bernard (2008) *Communication Skills for Health and Social Care*. Sage: London.

NHS Digital (2014) *Mental Health and Wellbeing in England. Adult Psychiatric Morbidity Survey. A National Statistics Publication*. NatCen Social Research and the Department of Health Sciences, University of Leicester:London and Leicester

Oliver, Michael (1996) *Understanding Disability. From Theory to Practice*. Macmillan: Basingstoke and London.

Pring, John (2019) 'User-led sector faces threat of extinction', *Disability News Service*, https://www.disabilitynewsservice.com/, 14 February 2019. Website accessed 19 February 2019.

Salman, Saba (2019) 'You can't rehabilitate someone back into society if they're locked away'. *The Guardian*, https://www.theguardian.com/society/2019/jan/16/rehab-centre-learning-disabilities-secure-units-community. Website accessed 21 March 2019.

Silberman, Steve. (2015) *Neurotribes. The Legacy of Autism and the Future of Neurodiversity*. Avery Publishing: New York.

Stossel, Scott (2013). *My Age of Anxiety. Fear, hope, dread, and the search for peace of mind*. Alfred A. Knopf: New York.

Scope (2019) https://www.scope.org.uk. Website accessed 17 March 2019.

Szasz, Thomas (1961, 1974) *The Myth of Mental Illness: Foundations of a Theory of Personal Conduct*. Harper & Row: New York.

Shakespeare, Tom (2014) 'Nasty, brutish and short', in Bickenbach, J., Felder, F., and Schmitz, B. (eds), *Disability and the Good Human Life*. Cambridge University Press: Cambridge.

Shaping our Lives (2019) Website accessed 19 March 2019. https://www.invo.org.uk/communities/invodirect-org/shaping-our-lives/

Townsend, P. (1962) *The Last Refuge: a survey of residential institutions and homes for the aged in England and Wales*. Routledge and Kegan Paul: London.

Union of the Physically Impaired Against Segregation (1976) *Fundamental Principles of Disability*. UPIAS: London.

Chapter 17

Communicating with children and young people

Present-day concerns about children and young people

Currently newspapers, television, radio and social media draw attention to concerns about children's well-being. Poverty still has an adverse effect on children and young people. Child abuse, including sexual abuse of children, is now more likely to be revealed rather than be hidden. Concerns about alcohol addiction, drug abuse, and delinquency are featured on television news and the internet. Adults worry about children's and young people's interest in social media, which can be a factor in emergent mental health problems. Yet these problems and concerns indicate that our society recognises the dangers of abuse and other behaviours and is now more sensitive and alert to children's difficulties than previously.

Communication with children and young people is a specialist skill

Communicating with children and young people is acknowledged as a specialist area of practice that requires specialist skills. For example, the British Association of Counselling and Psychotherapy (BACP) expects its registrant counsellors to undertake an extra period of training before beginning to practice with children and young people (BACP, 2018).

The recognition that practice with children and young people needs specialist knowledge and skillsis relatively recent. Traditionally, before the nineteenth century, children were not perceived as distinctive individuals, but as the possessions of their parents (BICE, 2019). Children had few legal rights of their own. Families were bound together by a patriarchal system under which married women owned no possessions: their income and property belonged to their husbands. No effective means of birth control was available, and wives were subservient to their husbands. Divorce was socially frowned upon and was difficult to obtain. Domestic abuse of women was not recognised or acknowledged. Over time, laws were changed to recognise the rights of women, children and young people, but changes did not occur instantly.

A look at the past: children's non-existent rights

Children were not entitled to receive an education or to learn how to read and write until the late nineteenth century (1870). Children worked long hours in fields, cotton mills, mines and in factories alongside their parents, if they were lucky. Otherwise they might become homeless, and be forced to beg on the streets or live in a punitive institution for the destitute, like the workhouse (Longmate, 2003). Poverty was a feature of their lives, and being poor or born out of wedlock led to punitive measures and moral blame (Heywood, 1959).

Gradually, humanitarian concern for orphaned, destitute and mistreated children led to changes in how they were treated. In the eighteenth and nineteenth centuries, Thomas Coram (the Foundling Hospital), Charles Dickens (*Oliver Twist*, 1836), Benjamin Waugh (NSPCC, 1873) and Dr. Barnardo, who established his first 'ragged school' in 1867, broadened awareness and created philanthropic organisations to help children. Welfare provision for children and young people improved, following social crises triggered by world events. During the First World War, the numbers of children born outside of marriage increased (Keating, 2008). After the war ended, Parliament passed the first Adoption Act for England and Wales that enabled children to be legally adopted. During the Second World War, children who were evacuated from London and other large cities to escape the bombing were placed in foster homes (Younghusband, 1964). The Kindertransport children (discussed in Chapter 14), who were sent to Britain to escape Nazi persecution, are another example of displaced children (Oppenheimer and Harris, 2008). These large-scale movements of children exposed the detrimental impacts of poverty and malnutrition on many evacuees. Although some were well cared for by their foster parents, others were mistreated and abused. This misuse of power and authority passed largely unnoticed until the death of Dennis O'Neill received national publicity. Dennis, aged 14, died in 1945 in miserable circumstances because of his foster parents' cruelty. His death led to a modern child care service (Stroud, 1965) being established. The new Children's Departments, founded in 1948, moved away from an emphasis on punishment and institutionalisation towards helping families stay together, or by placing children who could not live with their own parents with foster parents or adoptive parents.

Institutionalisation

Despite these changes, caring for delinquent, mistreated or abandoned children in institutions was a popular 'solution' until the 1970s. Many children whose parents were unable to provide care or who had been convicted of stealing or other misdemeanours were placed in boarding schools, children's homes and foster homes that were insufficiently regulated and inspected. Only in recent years has the hidden sexual abuse that went on in some institutions been revealed (Barter, 1999).

Traditional educational attitudes towards children

Attending school and learning to read and write were perceived as revolutionary in 1870 when laws were passed to provide compulsory primary education for children. A view prevailed that children were 'savages' who had to be 'tamed' through corporal punishment and derogatory criticism, and this attitude survived into the twentieth century.

Practice Example 17.1 *Soon after coming to live in the United Kingdom, I met three young female teachers, who discussed occasions when they 'had' to cane their pupils. These young women did not appear to be interested in exploring the reasons why a child might become naughty or attention-seeking, but saw their roles as whipping the children into submission.*

From 1944 to 1976, educational systems separated children into different groups via the '11-plus' examination, which identified the 20–25 per cent children deemed intelligent enough for an academic secondary education in grammar schools. Children who did not pass the 11+ received a 'secondary modern' education that provided few qualifications. Dividing children up by ability provided the economy with sufficient well-educated adults to teach in universities, fill the officer class of the armed services, administer the outposts of empire, and manage industrial concerns. The educational system was a tool of social policy and social engineering (Finch, 1984). Children who failed the 11+ believed themselves to be inferior.

> Practice Example 17.2 A group of mature students began their social work course, and shared their hopes and fears. Most of them entered the course without any previous formal academic qualifications but with years of experience working in social care. They began to admit their feelings of impending doom about the course, believing that they were 'stupid' because many years ago they failed the 11+ examination. A sense of inferiority was engrained within them. Their tutor spoke to them firmly and positively about their achievements over the years in an attempt to help them change their thinking about themselves. Eventually they found the courage to begin the course, and they gradually discovered that they did have the ability to pass the course.

Although the 11+ and other means of selective education still survive in some counties, the British educational system changed along with society itself, which now requires a better educated population to meet the demands of new employment opportunities. Society's changing nature led to the expansion of university degrees and college courses to meet contemporary demands for skills. Increased numbers of young people were able to complete university degrees successfully. The fallacy of the 11+ as a reliable predictor of future attainment was exposed (Spicker, 2019).

Health and communication

In the pre-antibiotic days, doctors were fearful that new born infants might contract a fatal infection or disease. Providing plenty of fresh air, feeding babies according to a strict schedule, and not handling a baby too much was the regime urged for new mothers by Dr Truby King, a leading paediatrician of the early twentieth century (Truby King, 1908, 1945). Feeding infants up to the age of six months at regular intervals with sterilised bottles and strictly measured 'baby formula' was a rigid routine, prompted by the fear of infection that might prove fatal. Not until antibiotics became widely available after the Second World War did Dr. Benjamin Spock urge parents to feed their babies on demand and pick up and hold their babies – a warmer kind of parenting which became the norm (Spock, 1946).

Before antibiotics became available, an unpopular but necessary health policy that negatively impacted on children's relationships with their parents was the strictly controlled limited visiting hours for hospitalised children. This policy was enforced when the fear of infection causing illness and death was paramount. Limiting hospital visiting hours was seen as a life-saving strategy. Consequently, visitors were not welcome in hospital wards. This separation could create a rift in the relationship between parent and child, but was required for health reasons.

> Practice Example 17.3 In the 1940s, a *two-year-old boy damaged his eye and eyelid when he fell against a door. He was rushed to hospital for a life-saving operation. Visiting hours were very restricted. When he was ready to come home from hospital after a week of not seeing his mother, she was very upset to hear him calling the ward nurse 'Mummy'.*

In the present day, under the National Health Service, general practitioners, practice nurses, children's nurses, midwives, paediatricians, public health practitioners, district nurses and health visitors work together to provide services that promote and maintain the health and well-being of adults, infants, children and young people. The Health Service also maintains well established multi-professional safeguarding services and committees. Parents generally perceive Health Service staff positively, in recognition of their dependence on and appreciation of the health care they receive. The Health Service's efforts have led to improved infant survival rates and a better quality of life for children and families.

Children's perceptions of personhood and authority

Children grow and learn from the people around them: parents, grandparents, other relatives, friends and neighbours, and for children in care, their foster parents or house parents. As they move towards adulthood, children hear their caregivers make statements about how they expect their children to behave. Traditional attitudes might include:

- 'Children should be seen and not heard'.
- 'Do as I say'.
- 'Don't argue!'
- 'Don't ask why, just obey!'

Some children become used to an absence of explanations, and not being expected to question, challenge, speak out or argue, but this kind of socialisation can damage their ability to ask for help when they reach adulthood.

> Practice Example 17.4 *A woman wanted to ask the district nurse for advice and help for her physical condition, but she felt frightened and uneasy. She thought that she would be criticised for needlessly asking for help. When she was a child, her mother had discouraged her from admitting anything was wrong and seeking help. Her mother's reactions stayed with her throughout adulthood, so that having to ask for help triggered fears of being rejected and criticised.*

The influence of attachment theory

Children's health and social care can be divided into two eras: pre-Bowlby and post-Bowlby. John Bowlby was a psychologist and psychoanalyst who researched early childhood development, and published his work on maternal deprivation and attachment in 1951. He argued that infants and young children who lacked the experience of close maternal care risked being unable to express affection and feelings of belonging.

These reactions were noticeable in infants who had been placed in residential nurseries from birth, or who had been neglected. Up until the mid-1960s, some local authorities provided residential nurseries for infants in care, and some of these were located a long distance from their parents' homes, so that visiting their children became very difficult. Bowlby's findings made a lasting difference and led to changes in child care and welfare policies. The realisation that infants and young children need to form bonds of attachment with their primary caregivers led to the closure of large children's homes and residential nurseries, and increased professional efforts to keep children with their birth parents, or if this was not possible, to place them for adoption or in long-term foster care.

Rights of the Child

Gradually, children gained recognition as individuals with human rights, not just as their parents' possessions. In 1924, the League of Nations published the Geneva Declaration which was the first recognition of children's rights and parents' responsibilities to provide suitable care. The United Nations Declaration of the Rights of the Child was issued in 1959, and it outlined ten rights: the right to

- equality
- special protection for physical, mental and social development
- a name and nationality
- adequate nutrition, housing, and medical services
- special education and treatment when the child has a physical or mental handicap
- parents' and society's love and understanding
- recreational activities and free education
- be among the first to receive relief in all circumstances
- protection against all forms of neglect, cruelty and exploitation
- be brought up in a spirit of understanding, tolerance, friendship among peoples, and universal brotherhood(United Nations, 1959)

Social services departments: power and authority

Social services departments are located within local authorities that employ social workers, occupational therapists, and social care workers to provide services to adults and children. Children's services include fostering, adoption, safeguarding, and supervision of children and families. In the 1940s and 1950s, social workers used a psycho-social casework method influenced by Freudian analytic theory in their interactions with children and parents (Hollis, 1964). The prevalence of psychoanalytical approaches has now faded, driven out first by growing concerns about child poverty, and then by the priority given to safeguarding children from physical, emotional and sexual abuse. Social work practice became more of a socio-legal endeavour designed to protect vulnerable children and adults from harm. Some parents began to perceive social workers as overly-authoritarian in their manner and wielding a dreaded power to take their children away from them.

Practice Example 17.7 As a counsellor, I became acquainted with parents who had been taken into care as children, and had experienced poverty, abuse, and addictions. Now they were adults, striving to be good parents to their children. I heard them express overwhelmingly negative views about social services, fearing social workers' power to remove their children, and saying they would never be able to trust what a social worker told them. Another painful aspect of some women's childhoods was their experience of having been sexually abused by a trusted male family member, the abuse subsequently being denied by their families, and then being accused of lying.

Exacerbating these feelings was their lack of knowledge about their childhood, why they were removed from their parents, and why they ended up in children's homes. Their memories of their childhood were often vague. They had been placed in healthy environments, but were not fully informed about their histories and their parents. They wanted to know what had happened to them. Although the practice of using life story books (discussed in Chapter 14) to help fill in gaps in knowledge is now widespread, some adults who had spent periods of their childhood in care feel angry and betrayed by not having sufficient knowledge or information about their early lives. These women who had spent much of their childhood in care may feel deterred from gaining access to the records of their time in local authority care by their fear of authority and the complex forms they are required to complete. As adults, they want to be in control, and learn about their previous life in care and the circumstances that led to them being taken into care. To reiterate the message of Chapter 7, information giving is an essential part of communicating with children and young people, and professional practitioners need to acquire skills for age-appropriate communication on these sensitive matters.

Countering the impact of historic policies and practices

Children who are subject to authoritarian regimes where they are criticised, scolded, and punished and/or abused at home, school, and with their peers will find it difficult to engage in open communication. They may seek to disguise their true feelings, retreat into silence, or else may 'act out' with periods of anger and destructiveness. This makes communication with them difficult. The professional practitioner needs to develop indirect strategies to 'get through' to the child and to enable the child to 'get through' to the practitioner. The first priority is to gain the trust of the child by being truthful, explaining your role, being consistent and reliable in your approach and contacts with the child, and showing an interest in them.

Another essential step is to become familiar with a range of child development theories and then draw on suitable theoretical approaches for different situations. Different theories provide clues for making sense of a child's communication at a particular stage of development. Each theory offers an explanation of chosen aspects of child development; some focus on social development, some on psychological development; others on emotional, cognitive, moral, or physical development. They reach different conclusions about different aspects of development. Sigmund Freud (1986), Carl Jung (1963), and Erik Erikson (1950, 1993) devised a range of theories about psycho-social development; John Watson (1925) and B.F. Skinner (1974) developed behavioural child development theories; Arnold Gesell (1943) studied maturational development; Jean Piaget (1971) published cognitive development theory; Albert Bandura researched social learning theory (1986), Lev Vygotsky (1978) explored socio-cultural development theory, Lawrence Kohlberg (1991) studied stages of moral development, and Abraham Maslow devised the *hierarchy of needs*, that portrayed human needs as a hierarchical ladder ascending towards *self-actualisation* (1954, 1970, 1987). But although these theories and others, when considered together, provide comprehensive theoretical overviews of many aspects of development, they do not necessarily help a practitioner learn how to communicate effectively.

> Practice Example 17. 5 *As a social worker and counsellor, I learned many different child development theories, social work theory, psychology and sociology, and this learning continued throughout my ongoing practice in social work and counselling both in the UK and USA. When I began writing this chapter, I reviewed my previous learning and experience of communication with children and young people, and realised that I had never been taught the basic principles of how to communicate. Whatever communication skills I learned were developed through experience 'on the job'.*

It is not wrong to learn from experience throughout one's professional life, but acquiring knowledge of the fundamental principles of communication is important from the start. This chapter does not have the space to explain every principle in detail, but aims to encourage practitioners' continued professional learning about communication. New communication concepts, theories, and techniques develop over time, and others fall from favour – that is why keeping learning up to date is essential.

Practitioners are likely to want to draw on more than one developmental theory, as well as knowledge acquired from their own practice, in order to communicate effectively with children and young people. Practitioners should do more than listen to what is said; they need to ask themselves: *what is not being said?* One-to-one verbal communication is not the only effective style of communication with children and young people. Non-verbal communication takes place, revealed by facial expressions, body language, and eye gaze. Practitioners need to observe the non-verbal communication of the child: eye gaze, expressions, physical movements, and their eagerness or reluctance to engage with a practitioner, and then ask themselves 'why?'

Different techniques of communication

Depending on their stages of development, children and young people may find communicating with a practitioner less stressful if they both engage in some shared activity. Rather than the practitioner asking complex questions while looking directly at a child, a better approach might be to play a game together, draw pictures, or play with small figures and building blocks to build a more relaxed relationship and stimulate more natural communication. Examples of shared activities feature in Ferguson's research (2014) about how social workers can use car journeys to communicate with children and families; and Ross et al.'s study (2009) about how practitioners use guided walks and car journeys as occasions for communication with children and young people.

Communication within groups can be effective with children and young people. Therapeutic group work encourages participants' individual communications within a group, and observes their interactions with others. Communicating as a member of a group can instil a sense of belonging and support when the group members learn to trust each other so that they can share their experiences without fear of bullying or rejection. Other organised groups for children and young people may be designed primarily for recreational purposes or child care rather than for therapeutic purposes (playgroups, nurseries, cub scouts, brownies, scouts, youth clubs, drama groups, musical groups, walking groups, sports clubs, and team sports), but participation in these recreational groups may also serve a therapeutic purpose for some children and young people. However, little enjoyment takes place when a child feels compelled to attend a group for which they have no aptitude. Some children excel at games and some do not; some children can sing and others cannot carry a tune. Some children enjoy handicrafts, others do not. Choosing activities carefully is essential and this requires knowledge of the individual child.

Different kinds of intervention with children and young people

Examples of intervention with children and young people that emphasise parent–child communication and positive development include:

- Head Start programmes, begun from 1965 in the USA, which provide early childhood education, health support, parental involvement and activities that stimulate parent/child communication with pre-school children from low-income families.
- Sure Start programmes, established in the UK from 1998, are patterned after Head Start programmes to provide young children with a good start in life. Although funding has been reduced, Sure Start children's centres continue to offer supportive programmes that encourage communication between young children and their parents.
- A therapeutic play programme called *Theraplay* is provided for young children and parents, often in children's centres. For example, Chilwell Children's Centre in Nottingham offers the Theraplay programme. Theraplay is a child and family therapy that aims to build attachment, self-esteem, and trust, and encourage 'joyful engagement' by focusing on four concepts – *structure, engagement, nurture*, and *challenge* – and by making positive connexions between children and parents/caregivers.
- The British Association of Social Workers (BASW) is promoting 'relationship-based social work' (Ingram and Smith, 2018). Relationship-based social work is affirmed as essential for achieving effective outcomes. Relationships are recognised as complex, needing practitioner awareness of 'self'. Ingram and Smith state that current practice cultures may lead to difficulties in practising in 'relational ways'. Their article, written from a Scottish perspective, suggests that a 'radical shift' is required for issues of power, agency, and status if relationships are truly to characterise practice. Perhaps a relational approach will in the future change the all-too-frequent authoritarian nature of communication with children and young people towards a style of communication that is more open and egalitarian. A practical difficulty will be the need for practitioners to develop more appropriate communication skills for practice with children and young people.
- Talking and Listening to Children (TLC) is a collaborative research project (http://www.talkingandlisteningtochildren.co.uk, 2019) funded by the Economic and

Social Research Council (ESRC). The project involves four universities: Sussex, Queen's Belfast, Edinburgh, and Cardiff, and aims to explore how social workers communicate with children; how social workers and children experience and understand these communications; identify the barriers to and enablers of effective communication; and develop resources to help attain improvements in communication.

- Gillian Ruch, Professor of Social Work at Sussex University, has launched a *Kitbag Campaign* to help social workers obtain and use interactive child-centred materials (including finger puppets, and feelings and emotions cards) to help their communications with children. A social worker could keep the material together in their Kitbag and take it with them when they meet with individual children. The British Association of Social Workers supports the Kitbag campaign. The concept of the Kitbag was developed by the Scottish educational charity International Futures Forum (http://www.iffpraxis.com/kitbag) which is planning to develop a 'community of practice' for practitioners who use this communication approach. At present, it is believed that only 20 per cent of social workers use interactive communication, and that employers are not providing social workers who want to use interactive communication methods with appropriate materials.

- Communication skills can benefit from learning about *social pedagogy* – a way of working with children, young people and adults that is practised widely in Europe where it is recognised as a form of social work. Social pedagogy is yet not widely well known in the United Kingdom, although Petrie (2011) and Cameron (2011) have written extensively about social pedagogy in the UK. The *social pedagogue* approach (Kaska, 2016) advocates holistic *social education* in informal settings rather than in a formal classroom. Social pedagogues use activities – games, music, and art – to develop opportunities for creative learning. Its *social education* approach aims to help children to reach their full potential, overcome social exclusion, and prevent and resolve social problems (Hamalainen, 2013). Social pedagogy emphasises relationships, self-reflection, empowerment, and a strength-based approach, similar to the strengths-based approach in social work (Saleebey, 2013). Influences on social pedagogy include the work of Rousseau (1712–1778) who sought to change society's understanding of childhood; Pestalozzi (1746–1827) who developed a 'discovery' approach to education; Dr. Barnardo (1845–1905) who developed children's homes and vocational opportunities for poor children; Maria Montessori (1870–1952), who developed a 'hands-on' self-directed learning method for children, and Korczak (1878–1942), a doctor who changed an orphanage into a participative, democratic 'children's republic' before perishing in the Holocaust. Social pedagogy's techniques help children and young people understand and observe behaviour in a non-judgemental way and make their own 'constructions of reality'. The social pedagogue's concept of the individual's *life-world* (Kraus, 2015) takes note of individual observations, experiences, and beliefs that help to form a person's growing sense of reality. Social pedagogy uses the concepts of *head* (logical thinking), *heart* (emotions and feelings) and *hands* (practical actions) to shape individual development (Pestalozzi, in Schmid, 1997). Because the social pedagogy approach is rooted in practice, a *practice apprenticeship* may provide an effective means of learning how to use the approach.

Summary

This chapter explored present-day concerns about children and young people, as well as traditional attitudes that denied children legal rights, education and institutionalised them when their parents were unable to care for them. The historic prevalence of poverty and moral blame affected their lives negatively. Gradual reform of children's services, prompted by new theoretical understanding, led to improvements in authoritarian regimes. Present-day communication with children and young people requires specialist practitioner skills to take account of children's stages of development and their level of communication skills. Current concerns about neglect and physical and sexual abuse challenge the ways professional practitioners communicate with children and young people. Communication skills are important for helping children and young people, particularly those who are in care, acquire knowledge of the events of their lives. It is hoped that a new emphasis on relationship-based work will lead to a less overtly authoritarian approach to communicating with children and young people. Petrie (2011) introduced principles of social pedagogy in her book about communication skills for working with children and young people. She summarises essential communication skills (pp. 168–171) as:

- listening
- not allowing your own feelings to distort the communication
- reflecting back your understandings of what has been said
- questioning others with care, and avoiding asking pointless or too many questions.
- speaking to individuals about unacceptable behaviour without challenging their self-esteem
- listening carefully so that you are able to take the other person's point of view, regardless of their age
- being aware of the part that feelings play in communication
- basing your communications on respect for the individual person

References

BACP (2018) *Therapy Today*. Accessed 20 March 2018, https://www.bacp.co.uk/media/2453/bacp-therapy-today-feb18.pdf

Bandura, A. (1986) *Social Foundations of Thought and Theory: A Social Cognitive Theory*. Prentice Hall: New York.

Barter, C. (1999) 'Practitioners' experiences and perceptions of investigating allegations of institutional abuse', *Child Abuse Review*, Volume 8, Issue 6, pp. 392–404.

Bowlby, J. (1953) *Child Care and the Growth of Love*. World Health Organisation: Geneva, Switzerland.

Corby, Brian (2006) *Child Abuse: Towards a Knowledge Base*. 3rd Edition: Open University Press: Maidenhead.

BICE (2019) *History of the Rights of the Child*. https://bice.org/en/history-rights-child/, Website accessed 28 March 2019.

Bowby, John (1953). *Child care and the growth of love*. Penguin Books: London.

Cameron, Claire and Moss, Peter (2011) (eds) *Social Pedagogy and Working with Children and Young People. Where Care and Education Meet*. Jessica Kingsley: London.

Dickens, Charles (1836) *Oliver Twist*. Bentley: London.

Erikson, E. (1950, 1993) *Childhood and Society*. W. W. Norton: New York.

Ferguson, H. (2010) 'Therapeutic Journeys: the car as a vehicle for working with children and families and theorizing practice', *Journal of Social Work Practice*, Volume 24, Issue 2, pp. 121–138.

Finch, F. (1984) *Education as Social Policy*Longmans: London.

Freud, S. (1986 edition) *The Essentials of Psycho-Analysis* (selected by Anna Freud). Penguin: London.

Gesell, A.And Ilg, F. (1943) *Infant and Child in the Culture of Today*. Harper and Row: New York.

Hamalainen, J. (2003) 'The concept of social pedagogy in the field of social work', *Journal of Social Work*, Volume 3, Issue 1, pp. 69–80.

Heywood, Jean S. (1959) *Children in Care*. Routledge: Abington.

Hollis, Florence (1964) *Casework. A Psychosocial Theory*. Random House: New York.

Ingram, R. and Smith, M. (2018) *Relationship-based –practice. Emergent themes in social work literature*. Insight 41. IRISS. http://www.iriss.org.uk/resources/insights/relationship-based-practice-em ergent-themes-social-work-literature. Website accessed 3 March 2019.

Jung, Carl (1963) *Memories, Dreams, Reflections*. Pantheon: New York.

Kaska, M. (2016) *Social Pedagogy. An Invitation*. Jacarinda Development: London.

Keating, Jenny (2008) *A Child for Keeps: The History of Adoption in England, 1918–45*. Palgrave Macmillan: Basingstoke.

Kohlberg, L. (1981) *Essays on Moral Development. Vol I The Philosophy of Moral Development*. Harper & Row. San Francisco, CA.

Koprowska, Juliet (2005, 2010) *Communication and Interpersonal Skills in Social Work*. 3rd Edition. Learning Matters Ltd: Exeter.

Korczak, J. (1939) *Playful Pedagogy*. Penguin: Warsaw.

Kraus, Bjorn (2015) 'The Life We Live and the Life We Experience: Introducing the Epistemological Difference between "Lifeworld" (Lebenswelt) and "Life Conditions" (Lebenslage)', *Social Work and Society International Online Journal*, Volume 13, Issue 2, p. 4.

Longmate, Norman (2003) *The Workhouse: A Social History*. Pimlico: London.

Maslow, A. (1954, 1970, 1987) *Motivation and Personality*. 3rd Edition, Harper and Row: New York.

Montessori, M. (1912) *The Montessori Method: Scientific paedagogy as applied to child education in 'the children's houses' with additions and revisions by the author*. Frederick Stokes Co: New York.

Oppenheimer, Deborah, and Harris, MarkJonathan (2008) *Into the Arms of Strangers: Stories of the Kindertransport*. Bloomsbury/St Martins: New York & London.

Petrie, Pat (1989, 2011) *Communication Skills for working with Children and Young People. Introducing Social Pedagogy*. 3rd Edition. Jessica Kingsley: London.

Piaget, J. (1971). 'The theory of stages in cognitive development', in D. R. Green, M. P. Ford, & G. B. Flamer, *Measurement and Piaget*. McGraw-Hill: New York.

Ross, N., Renold, E., Holland, S. and Hillman, A. (2009) 'Moving stories: using mobile methods to explore the everyday lives of young people in public care', *Qualitative Research*, Volume 9, pp. 605–623.

Saleebey, D. (2013) 'Introduction: Power in the people' in Saleebey, D., ed, *The Strength Perspective in Social Work Practice*. 6th Edition. Pearson Education: Upper Saddle River, NJ, pp. 1–24.

Schmid, Silvia (1997) 'Pestalozzi's Life Spheres', *Journal of the Midwest History of Education Society*, Cedar Falls, Iowa, University of Northern Iowa College of Education. Volume 23–24.

Skinner, B.F. (1974) *About Behaviorism*. Penguin/Random House: New York.

Spicker, Paul (2019) *Education and social policy. An Introduction to Social Policy*. http://spicker.uk/social-policy/education.htm. Website accessed 28 July 2019.

Spock, Benjamin (1946) *The Common Sense Book of Baby and Child Care*. Pocket Books, New York.

Stroud, John (1965) *An Introduction to the Child Care Service*. Longmans: London.

Talking and Listening to Children Project (TLC) (2019)http://www.talkingandlisteningtochildren. co.uk. Website accessed 8 March 2019.

Truby King, F. (1908, 1945) *Feeding and Care of Baby*. Oxford University Press: London.

The Kitbag (2019) International Futures Forum (http://www.iffpraxis.com/kitbag). Website accessed 8 March 2019.

United Nations (1959) *UN Declaration of the Rights of the Child*. UN: New York.

Vygotsky, L. (1978) *Mind in Society. The Development of higher psychological processes*. Harvard University Press: Cambridge, MA.

Watson, J.B. (1925) *Behaviorism*. W.W Norton: New York.

Waugh, B. (1873, 2010) *The Gaol Cradle, Who Rocks It?*Kessinger Publishing: Whitefish, MT, USA.

Younghusband, E. (1964) *Social Work and Social Change*Allen and Unwin: London.

Chapter 18

Professional development to improve your communication and interviewing skills

Prior learning and experience

Communication and interviewing are life skills, developed from childhood onwards. Prior achievements and experiences will influence how you select new learning about communication and interviewing. More than that, your previous learning helps to build your confidence in your own professional judgement.

For example, safeguarding of children and adults is a practice issue that spans the professions, with specific legislation and training required for all practitioners. When you accept a voluntary role of employment with an organisation, you have to undergo a DBS (Disclosure and Barring Service) check that scrutinises whether you have a previous criminal record, unspent convictions, cautions, reprimands and final warnings, and whether your name is on a list of individuals who are barred from fulfilling a particular occupation. Then, when appointed, you will have to complete mandatory training.

The area of safeguarding has been a public concern for several decades, but professional understanding and experience, as well as legislation, has expanded. When concerns about safeguarding first became part of protective legislation, the law focussed on protecting children and families, and was less concerned about neglect and cruelty to vulnerable adults. Over time, safeguarding legislation expanded to include adults. The history of safeguarding requirements illustrates how policy, practice and legislation continually change in response to newly identified concerns, and how these changes require practitioners to update their learning and practice. Their previous experiences contribute to their present practice, but these are tempered by new learning.

Safeguarding is not the only focus of change; all areas of practice continually develop new understandings of what constitutes good practice. Training increases practitioners' awareness of new requirements, but your previous professional experiences help you to communicate effectively with individuals and exercise professional judgement when you engage in safeguarding situations or other interactions with individuals. Previous learning and experience, including your communication and interviewing skills, provide a foundation for your ongoing learning and experience, and help you to further develop your professional judgement.

Professional development

A professional qualification is just the beginning. The essence of practising as a professional is your individual commitment to ongoing development through formal and informal learning, practice experience, selected reading, reflection, and supervision. Self-talk, peer support, and mentoring are supportive development activities. Undertaking different kinds of continuing professional development, listening to clients' feedback, and reflecting on practice are ways to build your practice wisdom. Your professional development should not be limited to your employer's training courses. Employers from time to time require you to update your knowledge of data protection, organisational procedures, safeguarding, and ethics (for example) but a curriculum vitae that lists only your employer's required training reveals a lack of commitment to your profession, which is more than being an employee.

Question: How do you choose your area of professional development?

Ideally, the choices you make will arise from your practice. Your interest might be prompted by wishing to discover possible strategies for situations that you encounter in your practice. The choices are up to you, and should not rely solely on a line manager requiring you to undertake a particular kind of training.

If you rely only on an employer or a professional regulator to decide what you need to know, you will be selling yourself short. Employers and regulators will specify their requirements, and you will need to comply, but your practice will always have wider boundaries. My own interest in loss and mourning arose from my previous professional and personal experiences. Questions formed in my mind as I observed people's different reactions to loss. I determined to learn more about the theoretical underpinnings of loss and mourning, and some of the new thinking about how individuals try to deal with their losses. I read relevant scholarly articles, sought out recent publications, attended two workshops on loss and mourning, and reflected on how I might draw on my new learning in my practice. I discussed my thoughts and reactions with my supervisor. There is still much for me to learn.

Continuing professional development for social workers in England

Social workers in England were previously regulated by two successive bodies: CCETSW (the Central Council for Education and Training in Social Work) and the GSCC (General Social Care Council), as well as the College of Social Work, which functioned as a professional body, but is now closed. Under CCETSW and the GSCC, social workers were exhorted to complete PQ (post qualifying) training courses.

- CCETSW approved awards and set up complex systems of regional consortia of employers and universities.
- The GSCC introduced a somewhat different system of complex PQ awards.
- The College of Social Work developed a ladder of Professional Capabilities for social workers, which, to this date, has survived under the aegis of the British Association of Social Workers (BASW, 2018).

You may be confused as you read this account – the previous systems were complex, and flawed. The CCETSW regional consortia each set their own expectations and did not succeed in achieving a national standard. Relatively few social workers undertook and completed PQ awards because of the cost and time implications.

The Health and Care Professions Council (HCPC) then assumed responsibility as the social work regulator in England. The Council's requirements for continuing professional development are flexible and cost effective, including learning by doing, practice studies, audits by service users, supervising staff or students, mentoring, teaching, undertaking research, gaining additional qualifications (HCPC, 2018). HCPC audits registrants' CPD activities regularly to ensure they retain their fitness to practice. In 2019 the social work profession in England will experience a change of regulator, moving from HCPC to the newly established regulatory body Social Work England, and it is not yet clear what that regulator will require for CPD.

Continuing professional development for social workers in Wales, Northern Ireland, and Scotland

Each of these countries has its own social work regulatory body and has experienced greater continuity in the requirements for continuing professional development. The 'Professional in Partnership' (PiP) in Northern Ireland has been successful in promoting and regulating a flexible, broadly based system of post qualifying studies that links practitioners, universities and employers for the purpose of promoting and providing a range of learning strategies.

Continuing professional development for health professions

Arts therapists, biomedical scientists, chiropodists/podiatrists, clinical scientists, dieticians, hearing aid dispensers, occupational therapists, operating department practitioners, orthoptists, paramedics, physiotherapists, practitioner psychologists, prosthetists/orthotists, radiographers, and speech and language therapists are regulated by the Health and Care Professions Council, and are subject to the same CPD requirements as social workers in England. The Nursing and Midwifery Council, the General Medical Council, the General Dental Council, and the General Pharmaceutical Council set their own CPD requirements. Doctors in the UK are registered with the General Medical Council, and must undergo periodic re-validation to ensure they are up-to-date. They choose appropriate CPD activities that demonstrate their fitness to practice, and are appraised.

Continuing professional development for counsellors

Counsellors are registered on voluntary registers that, sometimes, in my view, give the impression of competing with each others' standards. This competition deters efforts to establish counselling as a statutorily registered profession.

CPD requirements for counsellors expect practitioners to plan and keep a record of their chosen CPD activities – defined as any learning experience that can be used to broaden skills and competence. Feedback from people who use services should be an important element of CPD for all professions and this is easier to obtain when professional practitioners engage with a group of Experts by Experience who contribute to management and quality assurance systems. Counselling registration bodies apparently do not yet engage with clients' organisational networks to gather client feedback, making the views of clients about the quality of the counselling services they receive less easy to access than in other professions.

Questions and uncertainties about CPD will remain. Learning is ongoing and never completed. Whatever your profession, you will need to recognise the limits of your abilities and to remember that as a professional practitioner, you can develop and enhance your communication and interviewing skills through your practice experience, and through continuing professional development, reflection, peer consultation, and professional supervision.

Benner's stages of practice and the social work capabilities

You may wish to consider where to place yourself on Benner's stages of practice (1984). Benner's adaptation (1984) of the Dreyfus and Dreyfus model of skills acquisition suggested a staged ladder starting with a *novice practitioner*, progressing to *advanced beginner, competent practitioner, proficient practitioner*, and *expert practitioner*. The Dreyfus and Benner models represent efforts to understand and assist the development of skilled practitioners. The Benner stages indicate a slight correspondence with the social work Professional Capabilities Framework (PCF, BASW, 2018), which consists of four pre-qualifying levels of development (*point of entry to social work qualifying programmes, readiness for practice, end of first placement, end of last placement/completion of qualifying course*), followed by five levels: *newly qualified social worker; social worker; experienced social worker; advanced social worker; and strategic social worker.*

Attaining expertise

Eraut (2006, p. 8) argued that *expertise* requires different types of learning to acquire deliberative skills of critical analysis, interpretations of complex situations, and effective practice with other professionals and service users. Those different kinds of learning (formal education, training courses, reading, reflecting, and learning from others and your own experiences) are likely to be stimulated by different modes of study where you are a 'self-starter'. Through these activities, your assurance will increase, helping you to identify the strengths of your communication and interviewing skills as well as additional skills you wish to acquire.

The importance of research findings

A key question is: *how do I know when I am being helpful or unhelpful?* Efficacy of practice is affirmed by research into the outcomes of different interventions that draw on different theoretical approaches. Research on the effectiveness of contrasting strategies for communication and interviewing continues to be needed. An effective professional practitioner will try to keep up-to-date with new relevant research findings.

Hood (2018, pp. 126–127) offers an effective overview of research paradigms founded on different assumptions which influence the ways that new knowledge is shaped. *Positivist* research engages with social facts and laws and uses empirical methods drawn from the natural sciences. *Non-positivist* research includes *interpretivist* strategies that explore social reality and meaning; *realist* research explores causal mechanisms of events and behaviour; and *critical* research explores social structures of power, inequality, and emancipation. These different kinds of research require different research methods. Hood claims that academics, practitioners, and policy makers favour positivist studies that support searching for generalisable facts, whilst he argues for greater use of realist paradigms (Oliver, 2012) in social work research.

This discussion of research strategies could continue at length, but here it must suffice to remind practitioners of the importance of research, that practice needs to draw on relevant research findings, that each research paradigm has its strengths and limitations, that research findings can be useful for practice, but also that new research findings may modify or supersede long accepted methods. In summary, research is a dynamic activity whose findings practitioners must note and apply to shape their own practice.

Self-care

A practitioner may become engrossed in helping others, and then begin to neglect their own well-being. The BACP Ethical Framework (2018) contains a section on the practitioner's *care of self* as an essential part of sustaining good practice with clients. *Care of self* means taking responsibility for your own well-being, taking precautions to protect physical safety, monitoring and maintaining your psychological and physical health, ensuring that you are sufficiently resilient and resourceful to practice in ways that satisfy professional standards, and that you maintain a healthy balance between work and other aspects of life. These recommendations are not always easy to uphold.

> *Practice example 9.1 A social worker applied for a senior social work position with a local authority. The interview panel made deprecating remarks about the work of charities in the local area, implying that the charities had it easy and could pick and choose what they did. The panel boasted about their local authority social services: 'here we're working at the coal face – day-to-day practice is hard, and demands long hours and much time and effort, but it is "real" social work compared to the work of the charities.' The social worker subsequently discovered that, although the social services work was hard and demanding, their policies were flawed. He became critical of that local authority's frequent removal of children from their parents, their lack of interest in looked-after children's education, and the absence of partnership with voluntary organisations. He found it hard to accept the attitudes of his employing organisation which believed that its social workers were meant to work constantly 'at the coal face'. Exhaustion and staff burnout seemed a likely consequence of this attitude.*

> *Question:* How could this employer have prevented its professional practitioners from becoming overworked and disillusioned?

How can practitioners develop their communication and interviewing skills?

To become effective and maintain effectiveness, communication techniques can be used to gather useful, accurate knowledge and achieve clear factual understanding by listening carefully, using the 'restful pause' rather than non-stop volleys of words, and by recognising that 'less is more' – e.g. a few well-chosen words will achieve more understanding than a stream of lengthy complex sentences. Firing rapid questions turns a conversation into an inquisition. Using your *listening ear* helps to further good communication, and builds trust, a necessary quality for effective practice. Listening to the views of Experts by Experience can provide helpful feedback.

Building trust is achieved by revealing your humanity, using your facial expressions and gestures, tone of voice, and carefully chosen questions to form an effective working relationship with the person. The quality of empathy – not sympathy – helps foster a helpful professional relationship. Accepting the feelings of the person, when the person chooses to reveal them, is a therapeutic necessity, even when you disagree with the values expressed. Your non-judgemental manner signals acceptance of the person as he or she is, and is a precursor for helping the person find the courage to embark on their own journey of change.

As a professional practitioner, you should aim to be consistent and reliable. Your knowledge base will include an understanding of *use of self* and *therapeutic relationships*. Avoid telling the person what to do – giving orders – and instead make useful suggestions – *'have you thought about....?'* Interact therapeutically with the person who is angry, desperate, depressed, or hopeless, or perhaps feeling more than one of these emotions simultaneously. The person-centred approach (Rogers, 1961) can be used appropriately to sustain good practice in these situations. Recognising when a situation may pose a risk to yourself and others is a practice skill that prompts swift appropriate action to avert a crisis. These situations include the risk of violence, and the need to keep yourself and others safe.

How to select effective communication and interviewing strategies

Finally, this chapter offers some thoughts on how to 'put it all together', choose appropriate communication and interviewing skills, blend them, and use them in a suitable manner that proves beneficial to the people who seek help. As individuals, we live within social contexts – the social environments that influence our personal and social relationships. The individual forms a relationship with the society in which they live, and this relationship influences their life goals, values and moral and religious beliefs. Bronfenbrenner's ecological approach (1979, discussed in Chapters 2 and 6) draws attention to the different layers of relationships we experience: one-to one relationships (micro-level); family and friends relationships (meso-level), societal and employment relationships (macro-level) and relationships with the wider society (endo-level). Values, life goals, religious and spiritual beliefs inform powerful relationship structures within which an individual engages. Viktor Frankl's thinking about the *search for meaning* (2011, 1969, Chapter 6) suggests that this search constitutes a significant motivating force that shapes human behaviour. As well as dyadic, intimate relationships, the relationship of the individual self to the society in which they live helps to determine their life goals, values, and beliefs. The ways that individuals construct and reconstruct their understanding of themselves and others (Kelly, 1955; Neimeyer, 2009) indicate hope and opportunities for positive change.

The process of choosing appropriate techniques, using non-verbal communication and making use of information and questioning, illustrates the importance of practising the 'art' of communication (England, 1986, discussed in Chapter 4) by drawing on professional judgement, ethics and values, knowledge and experience. Skills and techniques for communication and interviewing should be chosen to fit the person's individuality and particular issues. The chosen technique must draw on the practitioner's strengths to maximise practice outcomes. A practitioner's growing expertise acquired through experience, ongoing learning, and support from professional supervision are crucial factors for learning how to communicate and interview effectively, and for developing relevant practice wisdom.

Summary

'Putting it all together' is not a science, but an art. The following statement (1 February 2017) by the late actor Sir John Hurt captures some of the essence of an 'art' – that as well as following an employer's processes, a practitioner should try to draw on their own professional judgement and creativity to choose how to proceed in a challenging practice situation. When asked by Geoff Andrew, a film critic and historian, how he turned in such good performances, Sir John said: *'The only way I can describe it is that I put everything I can into the mulberry of my mind and hope that it is going to ferment and make a decent wine. How that process happens, I'm sorry to tell you, I can't describe.'* This statement does not imply that the practitioner should throw away the rule book of accountable procedures, but rather, that he or she should begin to trust their own professional judgement and experience when communicating in sensitive situations.

References

BACP British Association of Counselling and Psychotherapy (2016) *Ethical Framework for the Counselling Professions*. BACP: Lutterworth.

BACP British Association of Counselling and Psychotherapy (2018) *Ethical Guidelines for Research in the Counselling Professions*. BACP: Lutterworth.

BASW (2018) *Professional Capabilities Framework* https://www.basw.co.uk/system/files/resources/Detailed%20level%20descriptors%20for%20all%20domains%20wi%20digital%20final1.pdf. Web site accessed 5 August 2018.

Benner, P. (1984) *From Novice to Expert*. Addison Wesley: Menlo Park, CA.

Bronfenbrenner, U. (1979) *The Ecology of Human Development*. Harvard University Press: Cambridge, MA.

Dreyfus, Stuart E. and Dreyfus, Hubert L. (February 1980). *A Five-Stage Model of the Mental Activities Involved in Directed Skill Acquisition*. California University Berkeley Operations Research Center: Berkeley, CA.

England, Hugh (1986) *Social Work As Art: Making Sense for Good Practice*. Allen & Unwin: London.

Eraut, Michael (2006) 'Professional Knowledge and Learning at Work', *Knowledge, Work &Society - Savoir, Travail et Société*, Volume 3, Issue 4, pp. 45–62.

Frankl, V. (2011, 1969) *Man's Search for Ultimate Meaning*. Basic Books: Cambridge, MA.

Health and Care Professions Council (2018) *Continuing Professional Development Activities*. www.hcpc-uk.org/registrants/cpd/activities/. Website accessed 4 August 2018.

Hood, Rick (2018) *Complexity in Social Work*. Sage: London.

Hurt, John (2017) 'The Mulberry of My Mind' https://www.brainyquote.com/quotes/john_hurt_191406. Website accessed 1 September 2018.

Kelly, G.A. (1955*) The Psychology of Personal Constructs*. Routledge: New York.

Neimeyer, Robert A. (2009) *Constructivist Psychotherapy*. Routledge: London.

Oliver, Caroline (2012) 'Critical Realist Grounded Theory: A New Approach for Social Work Research', *The British Journal of Social Work*, Volume 42, Issue 2, 1 March 2012, pp. 371–387.

Rogers, C. R. (1961) *On Becoming a Person*. Constable: London.

Chapter 19

Summarising key messages

- Chapter 1 established that the book is written for **professional practitioners and students of social work, counselling and the health professions**, introduced the book's aims, objectives, key themes, and organisational structure, provided synopses of the content, and discussed the importance of acquiring practice wisdom and exercising professional judgement in day-to-day practice.
- Chapter 2 discussed **persons who use services**, *intersectionality* (Collins and Bilge, 2016), the phases of effective communication, building trust, the seminal research that introduced ideas about personhood (Rogers, 1961) and relationships (Biestek, 1992, 1957), as well as concepts of active listening, personal and social contexts of communication, and shared humanity. The chapter explored how each profession uses different terminology to describe a person at the receiving end of a professional communication and considered the contributions of service users who are Experts by Experience (Beresford, 2016).
- Chapter 3 discussed **professional practitioners and their roles**, changing service user perceptions of practitioners, how social contexts influence communication, similarities and differences in communication, paternalistic, medical, social, participatory, and constructive models of communication, therapeutic relationships, rapport, empathy, different cultural and ethnic identities, essential skills, suggested protocols for communication, the art of practice, how changing service delivery contexts influence communication styles and why these different styles ebb and flow in popularity.
- Chapter 4 discussed how to choose **different communication approaches**, understand and use a repertoire of formal, informal, and group communication, give and receive information, identify how professional status hinders communication, recognise how service user and patient groups have changed the nature of professional communication, perceive communication as *heart–soul–emotion* and *head/mind/reason*, acknowledge the changing uses of relationships, the importance of reflection, the implicit and explicit use of power, and the art of practice.
- Chapter 5 discussed **interviewing skills for different purposes** using different interviewing styles, conducting an interview, being the interviewee, interviewing service users/clients/patients, group interviews, avoiding disillusionment with the process, professional power structures, Equal Opportunities legislation and procedures, and the contribution of Experts by Experience to interviewing processes.
- Chapter 6 discussed **conceptual bases for communication and interviewing in different practice situations**, including personal and social contexts that influence

communication, the search for meaning, construction and reconstruction of meaning, cognitive approaches, communication for specific professional roles, factors that help and hinder well-being, an ecological counselling approach, personal narratives, on-the-spot counselling, crisis intervention, attachment, loss, and mourning.

- Chapter 7 discussed **information giving** as a form of communication that provides individuals with a range of strategies for addressing their problems, and promotes choice, confidence, and assertiveness.
- Chapter 8 discussed **ethical concerns** for communication and interviewing, how new ethical concerns arise, and how practice changes in response to these concerns, how *intersectionality* influences ethics, conflicts of interest, shared confidentiality, commonalities and differences in ethical codes, ethical research issues, personhood and non-judgemental attitudes, and the importance of professional judgement and supervision.
- Chapter 9 discussed **communication and interviewing in different organisational contexts**, how to communicate effectively across professional boundaries and value others' contributions, organisational size and structures, issues of multi-professional teams, multi-professional practice, systems for recording data, bureaucracy, information technology and communication, and the demands of personalisation on practitioners' communication.
- Chapter 10 explored issues of communicating with **technology, computers, and artificial intelligence**, including the use of logarithms, power and control, unwitting bias and errors, and reasons why the use of technology may need more scrutiny. The roles of professional practitioners in using technology are discussed.
- Chapter 11 discussed **additional methods and approaches** for effective communication and interviewing, with a focus on how a practitioner can choose and combine different approaches, make decisions in new and challenging situations, rely on their professional judgement, and overcome possible blockages in communication. The chapter discussed communication with individuals who have mental health issues, diabetes, addictions, and obesity.
- Chapter 12 discussed how professional practitioners can communicate with people who face **situations of loss**. The chapter discussed different kinds of loss: death, but also loss of relationships, physical capacity, and financial security. The chapter reviewed different theories of loss and mourning, and discussed the kinds of support that practitioners might offer.
- Chapter 13 discussed **domestic violence** and communication, tracing the history of how domestic violence first became recognised and the helping responses. The work of women's refuges, issues about perpetrators of domestic violence, and different kinds of effective help are examined.
- Chapter 14 discussed the therapeutic use of **life stories** and **biographical approaches** for communicating with both children and adults. Professional practitioners can communicate collaboratively with their clients to construct the life story, and this can be helpful for individuals whose previous lives have been turbulent. This method of communication can help individuals begin to plan a new future after they have reviewed their past.
- Chapter 15 discussed **communication with older people,** and explored the different experiences of older people and how they are often stereotyped by society. The chapter sought to establish non-ageist communication and explored how communication with older people can avoid stereotypical negative assumptions about old age.

- Chapter 16 explored issues to consider when **communicating with people with a mental health issue, a physical impairment or learning difficulties,** including the history of neglect and institutionalisation, changing social policies, community care, the social model of disability, and the role of Experts by Experience. Communication requires accepting and valuing their contributions. The chapter discussed the importance of language for establishing good communication.
- Chapter 17 discussed communication with **children and young people,** first exploring traditional authoritarian attitudes towards children and their care, and how these attitudes have changed. Specialist skills of communicating with children and young people with life story books and play therapy strategies were discussed, including the work of children's centres.
- Chapter 18 discussed taking responsibility for **professional development** and seeking to continuously improve your communication and interviewing skills through self-reflection, new techniques, continued learning, and supervision. The chapter discussed the important of *self-care* for professional practitioners.
- **Chapter 19** summarises the book's **content and main themes**, and invites professional practitioners to further develop their skills and knowledge of communication.

Some final considerations

Throughout, the book has pursued its objectives of encouraging practitioners to draw on personal and social contexts to enhance their professional judgement, to value the importance of constructing and reconstructing meaning, searching for meaning, understanding situations of loss, developing practice wisdom relevant to their profession, exercising professional judgement, and applying communication and interviewing skills within multi-professional contexts. As the book reaches its conclusion, I reiterate some themes that can help a practitioner think through the complexity of communication and interviewing, improve their communication and interviewing skills, and develop an effective style of their own.

- Consider and combine the separate components of *the person who uses services+ the practitioner + the particular issue + ethical considerations + context + methods and approaches.*
- Integrate your practice skills through your awareness of a *mix of social and psychological influences* on an individual's behaviour and well-being.
- Remember that practitioners communicate increasingly within multi-*professional contexts.*
- Provide *clear information* for professional communication, and avoid professional jargon, acronyms, and discussion that are unintelligible to persons who receive services.

An important message for practitioners is to understand how patient/service user/client groups modify the use of professional power in communication. Each profession is now expected to take note of the views and feedback of persons who use services. Their participation modifies the use of professional power in communication and interviewing. Communication with clients, patients, and people who use services should reflect the new kinds of partnerships between them and professional practitioners.

Choosing your own individual strategies for communication and interviewing

Your task as a practitioner is to choose appropriate individual strategies for practising effectively in particular situations. Your strategies are likely to include:

Introducing yourself

- Introduce yourself and any others present by name and professional role; explain why you and they are present, and the purpose of the meeting. Speak slowly and clearly, use plain English, avoid jargon, professional acronyms, colloquialisms and stereotyped cultural assumptions; ensure that the person can hear you, and if the person does not understand English, arrange for an interpreter; use open-ended questions and ensure that your communication has been understood.

Communicating clearly

- Communicate clearly to each individual, explain the scope and limits of confidentiality and what happens to shared information; then recapitulate and summarise your discussion.

Conveying acceptance of the person

- Convey acceptance of the person and build trust with a look, a nod, or a restful pause, rather than by torrents of words; remember that 'less is more': a few words can make a more positive impact than a flow of many words that overwhelm the person; and maintain reliability and consistency by being prepared and turning up on time.

Enabling the person at the receiving end of professional communication to respond

- Encourage questions from the person who uses services. Inform the person(s) about your organisation's complaints/appeal process; invite the person's comments and ask for their views.

Summing up

This book cannot expect to cover all aspects of communication and interviewing in depth. The book has attempted to develop overall understanding but has also sought to stimulate your interest, and encourage you to explore some topics further through selective reading, supervision, and reflection. Developing your communication and interviewing skills is an ongoing task, and your achievement will become evident as you make a determined effort to acquire more knowledge and experience and to think more deeply about how you can improve your practice.

References

Biestek, F. (1992, 1957) *The Casework Relationship*. Routledge: London.
Beresford, P. (2016) *All Our Welfare: Towards Participatory Social Policy*. Policy Press: London.
Collins, Patricia Hill and Bilge, Sirma (2016) *Intersectionality*. Polity Press: Cambridge.
Rogers, C. R. (1961) *On Becoming a Person*. Constable: London.

Index

Made in the USA
Las Vegas, NV
09 February 2022

43482902R00118